15-MINUTE DIABETIC DIET COOKBOOK EASY RECIPES FOR BEGINNERS

Complete guide to 2000-days of tasty , quick and easy diabetic-friendly recipes to control blood sugar, perfect for prediabetic, newly diagnosed and type 2 diabetes, with a 31-day meal plan

Nathan Wendy

Table of Contents

COPYRIGHT © 2023

CHAPTER ONE

Introduction to the 15-Minute Diabetic Diet Cookbook

The 15-Minute Diabetic Diet Cookbook serves as a beacon of hope for individuals managing diabetes who often find themselves strapped for time. In today's fast-paced world, balancing health and convenience can be a daunting task, particularly for those navigating the complexities of dietary management. This cookbook is a testament to the idea that healthy eating need not be time-consuming or arduous. Through a meticulously curated collection of recipes, it empowers individuals with diabetes to reclaim control of their health without sacrificing precious time.

Welcome to Quick and Easy Diabetic Cooking

In the realm of diabetic cooking, convenience is often synonymous with compromise. Many pre-packaged "diabetic-friendly" options flood the market, promising convenience but delivering subpar nutritional value. This subchapter serves as a warm invitation to a new approach—one that prioritizes both speed and health. Quick and easy diabetic cooking is not about cutting corners; it's about strategic planning and clever execution. From vibrant salads to hearty soups, each recipe in this cookbook has been carefully crafted to deliver maximum flavor and nutrition in minimal time.

Within this subchapter, readers are introduced to the ethos of quick and easy cooking. It's about embracing simplicity without sacrificing taste or nutrition. The recipes featured in this cookbook are designed to streamline the cooking process, allowing individuals with diabetes to enjoy delicious meals without the stress of extensive preparation. Whether you're a seasoned chef or a novice in the kitchen, this section welcomes you with open arms, inviting you to embark on a culinary journey that prioritizes both health and convenience.

Benefits of 15-Minute Meals for Diabetes Management

The benefits of 15-minute meals extend far beyond mere convenience. For individuals managing diabetes, time is of the essence. Blood sugar levels fluctuate throughout the day, requiring careful monitoring and timely intervention. Traditional meal preparation often demands hours of laborious cooking, leaving little room for spontaneity or flexibility. In contrast, 15-minute meals offer a lifeline for busy individuals, providing a quick and easy solution to the perpetual dilemma of time versus health.

One of the primary benefits of 15-minute meals for diabetes management is their ability to streamline the cooking process without compromising nutritional integrity. By leveraging simple ingredients and efficient cooking techniques, these meals deliver a powerful combination of flavor, convenience, and health benefits. Moreover, the rapid turnaround time ensures that individuals can enjoy freshly prepared meals without the need for extensive planning or preparation.

Another advantage of 15-minute meals is their adaptability to various dietary preferences and restrictions. Whether you follow a vegetarian, vegan, or omnivorous diet, there are plenty of options available to suit your needs. Additionally, these meals can easily accommodate food allergies and sensitivities, making them suitable for individuals with diverse nutritional requirements.

From a psychological standpoint, the immediacy of 15-minute meals can have a profound impact on adherence to dietary guidelines. Many individuals with diabetes struggle with feelings of overwhelm and frustration when faced with the prospect of complex meal preparation. By offering a quick and easy alternative, this cookbook empowers individuals to take control of their health without succumbing to feelings of deprivation or restriction.

In summary, the benefits of 15-minute meals for diabetes management are multifaceted. They offer a practical solution to the time constraints faced by busy individuals while simultaneously promoting optimal health and well-being.

Tips for Success: Kitchen Efficiency and Meal Planning

Efficiency is the cornerstone of successful meal planning, especially for individuals managing diabetes. In a world where time is a precious commodity, mastering the art of kitchen efficiency can make all the difference. This section offers practical tips and strategies for streamlining the cooking process and maximizing productivity in the kitchen.

One of the first steps towards kitchen efficiency is establishing a well-organized workspace. This involves decluttering countertops, organizing utensils and ingredients, and ensuring that essential cooking tools are readily accessible. By creating a clear and clutter-free environment, you can minimize distractions and optimize workflow.

Meal planning is another crucial component of kitchen efficiency, particularly for individuals with diabetes. By prepping ingredients in advance and planning meals for the week ahead, you can save time and reduce stress during busy weekdays. This cookbook provides a wealth of meal planning resources, including customizable meal plans, shopping lists, and prep-ahead tips to help you stay on track with your dietary goals.

In addition to meal planning, mastering basic cooking techniques can significantly enhance kitchen efficiency. From knife skills to time-saving cooking methods, there are countless ways to streamline the cooking process and minimize prep time. This section offers step-by-step instructions and helpful illustrations to guide you through essential cooking techniques, ensuring that you can whip up delicious meals in record time.

Finally, don't underestimate the power of batch cooking and leftovers. By preparing large batches of meals and portioning them into individual servings, you can save time and energy throughout the week. Leftovers can be repurposed into creative new dishes or enjoyed as quick and easy meals on busy days. With a little creativity and planning, you can turn leftovers into a valuable resource for kitchen efficiency.

In conclusion, kitchen efficiency is essential for success in diabetic cooking. By implementing the tips and strategies outlined in this section, you can streamline the cooking process, save time, and enjoy delicious meals without the stress of extensive preparation.

CHAPTER TWO

Essential Tools and Ingredients for Quick Cooking

In the realm of quick cooking, having the right tools and ingredients at your disposal can make all the difference between a stressful mealtime scramble and a smooth culinary experience. This subchapter delves into the essential tools and ingredients that are indispensable for preparing delicious meals in record time while managing diabetes.

Must-Have Kitchen Tools for Fast Cooking

Efficiency in the kitchen starts with having the right tools for the job. While fancy gadgets and gizmos abound, there are a few essential kitchen tools that every home cook should have in their arsenal, especially when aiming for quick cooking.

1. **Chef's Knife**: A sharp chef's knife is the workhorse of the kitchen. It allows for precise slicing, dicing, and chopping, making quick work of ingredients like vegetables, fruits, and proteins.

2. **Cutting Board**: A sturdy cutting board provides a safe and stable surface for chopping ingredients. Opt for one that is large enough to accommodate your chopping needs without crowding.

3. **Nonstick Skillet or Saute Pan**: A nonstick skillet or saute pan is essential for cooking proteins, stir-fries, and quick sautes without the hassle of food sticking to the pan.

4. **Instant-Read Thermometer**: An instant-read thermometer ensures that proteins are cooked to the proper temperature without overcooking. This tool is especially useful for quick-cooking meats like chicken breasts or fish fillets.

5. **Vegetable Peeler**: A vegetable peeler makes quick work of peeling vegetables and fruits, saving time and effort in meal preparation.

6. **Immersion Blender or Food Processor**: An immersion blender or food processor is invaluable for quickly pureeing soups, sauces, and dressings without the need for transferring ingredients to a separate appliance.

7. **Microwave Oven**: While not a traditional kitchen tool, a microwave oven can be a lifesaver for quick cooking. It can rapidly heat ingredients, thaw frozen foods, and even cook entire meals in a fraction of the time required for conventional methods.

8. **Measuring Cups and Spoons**: Accurate measuring is essential for successful cooking, especially when following recipes. Invest in a set of measuring cups and spoons to ensure precise ingredient proportions.

9. **Timer**: A reliable timer helps you keep track of cooking times and prevents dishes from overcooking or burning. Most kitchen timers are inexpensive and easy to use, making them a must-have for quick cooking.

10. **Mixing Bowls**: A set of mixing bowls in various sizes is essential for mixing ingredients, marinating meats, and

storing leftovers. Opt for bowls that are durable, lightweight, and easy to clean.

By equipping your kitchen with these essential tools, you'll be well-prepared to tackle any recipe with ease, efficiency, and confidence.

Essential Ingredients for 15-Minute Diabetic Meals

The key to quick cooking lies in having a well-stocked pantry and refrigerator. With a few essential ingredients on hand, you can whip up delicious meals in a matter of minutes, even when time is tight. This section explores the essential ingredients that form the foundation of 15-minute diabetic meals.

1. **Fresh Vegetables**: Fresh vegetables are the cornerstone of healthy cooking. Stock up on versatile options like spinach, kale, broccoli, bell peppers, and tomatoes, which can be incorporated into a wide range of dishes.

2. **Lean Proteins**: Lean proteins are essential for balanced meals that keep blood sugar levels stable. Opt for options like skinless chicken breast, turkey breast, fish, tofu, and legumes, which cook quickly and provide essential nutrients without excess fat or calories.

3. **Whole Grains**: Whole grains are rich in fiber and complex carbohydrates, which help regulate blood sugar levels and

promote satiety. Keep quick-cooking options like quinoa, brown rice, whole wheat pasta, and oats on hand for easy meal preparation.

4. **Healthy Fats**: Healthy fats add flavor and richness to meals while providing essential nutrients and promoting heart health. Incorporate sources like avocado, olive oil, nuts, and seeds into your recipes in moderation for optimal flavor and nutrition.

5. **Herbs and Spices**: Herbs and spices are the secret weapons of quick cooking, adding depth, complexity, and flavor to dishes without excess calories or sodium. Keep a variety of options on hand, such as garlic, ginger, basil, oregano, cumin, and chili powder, to elevate your culinary creations.

6. **Low-Sodium Broth or Stock**: Low-sodium broth or stock serves as the base for soups, stews, and sauces, infusing dishes with rich flavor without the need for excessive salt. Stock up on both vegetable and chicken broth for maximum versatility.

7. **Canned Beans and Tomatoes**: Canned beans and tomatoes are pantry staples that can be quickly incorporated into a variety of dishes, including soups, salads, and stir-fries. Opt for low-sodium varieties whenever possible and rinse canned beans before using to reduce sodium content.

8. **Citrus Fruits**: Citrus fruits like lemons, limes, and oranges add brightness and acidity to dishes, balancing flavors and enhancing taste. Keep a few on hand for zesting, juicing, and garnishing your culinary creations.

9. **Low-Sodium Soy Sauce or Tamari**: Low-sodium soy sauce or tamari adds savory umami flavor to dishes without excess sodium. Use it sparingly to season stir-fries, marinades, and sauces, adding depth and complexity to your recipes.

10. **Low-Sugar Condiments**: Condiments like mustard, vinegar, hot sauce, and salsa are essential for adding flavor to dishes without extra calories or sugar. Look for options labeled "low-sugar" or "no added sugar" to keep blood sugar levels in check.

By keeping these essential ingredients on hand, you'll be well-equipped to whip up delicious and nutritious meals in a flash, even on the busiest of days.

Smart Grocery Shopping and Ingredient Substitutions

Smart grocery shopping is the key to success when it comes to quick cooking. By planning ahead and making strategic choices at the grocery store, you can streamline meal preparation and ensure that you always have the ingredients you need on hand. This section offers practical tips for efficient grocery shopping and creative ingredient substitutions to accommodate dietary preferences and restrictions.

1. **Plan Ahead**: Before heading to the grocery store, take inventory of your pantry, refrigerator, and freezer to identify what ingredients you already have on hand and what you need to purchase. Create a shopping list based on planned meals for the week ahead, taking into account any special dietary considerations or preferences.

2. **Shop the Perimeter**: When navigating the aisles of the grocery store, focus on the perimeter, where fresh produce, lean proteins, and dairy products are typically located. This will help you prioritize whole, unprocessed foods and minimize exposure to tempting processed snacks and sweets.

3. **Read Labels**: Take the time to read food labels carefully, paying attention to ingredients, nutritional information, and serving sizes. Look for options with minimal added sugars, sodium, and unhealthy fats, opting instead for whole, nutrient-dense foods whenever possible.

4. **Choose Convenience Wisely**: While convenience foods can be a time-saving option, they often come with a hefty price tag in terms of added sugars, sodium, and preservatives. When selecting convenience items like pre-cut vegetables,

frozen meals, or canned soups, opt for options with minimal added ingredients and preservatives.

5. **Consider Seasonality**: Embrace seasonal produce whenever possible, as it tends to be fresher, more flavorful, and more budget-friendly than out-of-season options. Visit farmers' markets or join a community-supported agriculture (CSA) program to access a wide variety of locally grown fruits and vegetables.

6. **Stock Up on Staples**: Keep your pantry stocked with essential staples like whole grains, canned beans, nuts, seeds, herbs, and spices, which can be used to create a wide range of quick and easy meals. This will allow you to whip up nutritious dishes on short notice without the need for a trip to the grocery store.

7. **Embrace Imperfection**: Flexibility is key when it comes to smart grocery shopping. If a specific ingredient is unavailable or out of season, don't be afraid to improvise and make substitutions based on what you have on hand. Experimenting with new ingredients and flavor combinations can lead to exciting culinary discoveries.

8. **Minimize Food Waste**: Be mindful of food waste when grocery shopping, and strive to use up perishable ingredients before they spoil. Plan meals that incorporate leftovers and

use up odds and ends in creative ways to minimize waste and maximize efficiency in the kitchen.

By adopting these smart grocery shopping strategies and embracing ingredient substitutions, you can streamline meal preparation, minimize waste, and ensure that you always have the ingredients you need to whip up delicious and nutritious meals in a flash.

CHAPTER THREE

Breakfasts Ready in 15 Minutes or Less

Breakfast is often hailed as the most important meal of the day, yet it's also the one that tends to get neglected when time is short. This subchapter explores the art of preparing quick and delicious breakfasts that can be ready in 15 minutes or less, making it easy to start your day on the right foot, even when time is tight.

Quick and Nutritious Breakfast Ideas

When it comes to quick breakfasts, simplicity is key. This section offers a variety of nutritious breakfast ideas that can be prepared in a matter of minutes, ensuring that you can fuel your body with the energy it needs to tackle the day ahead.

1. **Greek Yogurt Parfait**: Layer Greek yogurt with fresh fruit, nuts, seeds, and a drizzle of honey for a quick and satisfying breakfast that's packed with protein, fiber, and essential nutrients.

2. **Whole Grain Toast with Nut Butter**: Top whole grain toast with your favorite nut butter and sliced banana or berries for a hearty and satisfying breakfast that provides a balance of carbohydrates, protein, and healthy fats.

3. **Vegetable Omelet**: Whip up a quick vegetable omelet by sautéing your favorite veggies, such as spinach, bell peppers, onions, and mushrooms, then folding them into beaten eggs and cooking until set. Serve with whole grain toast for a complete meal.

4. **Avocado Toast**: Mash ripe avocado onto whole grain toast and top with sliced tomatoes, a sprinkle of salt and pepper, and a drizzle of balsamic glaze for a simple yet satisfying breakfast that's rich in healthy fats and fiber.

5. **Smoothie Bowl**: Blend together frozen fruit, leafy greens, Greek yogurt, and a splash of milk or juice until smooth, then pour into a bowl and top with your favorite toppings, such as granola, nuts, seeds, and coconut flakes, for a refreshing and nutrient-packed breakfast option.

6. **Breakfast Burrito**: Fill a whole grain tortilla with scrambled eggs, black beans, diced vegetables, and a sprinkle of cheese, then roll it up and enjoy a portable and protein-rich breakfast that's perfect for busy mornings.

7. **Chia Seed Pudding**: Mix together chia seeds, milk, and a touch of sweetener, then let it sit in the refrigerator overnight to thicken. In the morning, top with fresh fruit, nuts, and a drizzle of honey for a nutritious and satisfying breakfast that requires minimal effort.

8. **Whole Grain Cereal with Milk**: Opt for a high-fiber, low-sugar whole grain cereal and top it with milk or a plant-based alternative for a quick and convenient breakfast that's rich in vitamins, minerals, and fiber.

9. **Egg Muffins**: Preheat the oven to 350°F and grease a muffin tin. Fill each muffin cup with beaten eggs and your choice of vegetables, cheese, and cooked protein, then bake for 15-20 minutes until set. Enjoy egg muffins hot or cold for a portable and protein-packed breakfast option.

10. **Fruit and Nut Bars**: Choose a high-protein, low-sugar fruit and nut bar for a convenient breakfast option that you can enjoy on the go. Look for options made with whole food ingredients and minimal added sugars for optimal nutrition.

By incorporating these quick and nutritious breakfast ideas into your morning routine, you can ensure that you start your day off right with a balanced and satisfying meal that provides the energy and nutrients you need to thrive.

Breakfast Smoothies and Overnight Oats

Smoothies and overnight oats are two breakfast staples that are perfect for busy mornings. This section explores how to prepare these quick and convenient breakfast options, ensuring that you can enjoy a nutritious meal even when time is short.

1. **Breakfast Smoothies**: To prepare a breakfast smoothie, simply combine your favorite fruits, leafy greens, Greek yogurt or protein powder, and a liquid base such as milk, juice, or water in a blender. Blend until smooth, then pour into a glass and enjoy immediately. Smoothies are highly customizable, so feel free to experiment with different flavor

combinations and add-ins to suit your taste preferences and nutritional needs.

2. **Overnight Oats**: Overnight oats are a simple and convenient breakfast option that can be prepared the night before and enjoyed cold or heated up in the morning. To make overnight oats, combine rolled oats with milk or a plant-based alternative, Greek yogurt or chia seeds, and your choice of sweetener and flavorings in a jar or container. Stir well, then cover and refrigerate overnight. In the morning, top with fresh fruit, nuts, seeds, or nut butter for added flavor and texture, then enjoy a delicious and nutritious breakfast without any hassle.

Smoothies and overnight oats are both highly versatile and can be customized to suit your taste preferences and dietary needs. Whether you prefer a fruity smoothie or a creamy bowl of oats, these quick and convenient breakfast options are sure to satisfy your hunger and fuel your body for the day ahead.

Simple Egg Recipes for Busy Mornings

Eggs are a versatile and nutritious breakfast option that can be prepared in a variety of ways in just a matter of minutes. This section explores some simple egg recipes that are perfect for busy mornings when you need a quick and satisfying meal.

1. **Scrambled Eggs**: To make scrambled eggs, crack eggs into a bowl and whisk together with a splash of milk or water until

well combined. Heat a nonstick skillet over medium heat and add the beaten eggs, stirring gently with a spatula until they are cooked to your desired consistency. Season with salt and pepper, then serve hot with whole grain toast or fresh fruit for a balanced and satisfying breakfast.

2. **Fried Eggs**: To fry eggs, heat a nonstick skillet over medium heat and add a small amount of butter or oil. Crack eggs into the skillet and cook until the whites are set and the yolks are still runny, about 2-3 minutes. Carefully flip the eggs using a spatula and cook for an additional 1-2 minutes until the yolks are cooked to your desired consistency. Serve hot with whole grain toast or sautéed vegetables for a quick and nutritious breakfast option.

3. **Egg Sandwich**: To make an egg sandwich, scramble or fry eggs according to your preference and place them on a whole grain English muffin or sandwich thin. Top with sliced avocado, tomato, spinach, or cheese, then season with salt, pepper, and any other desired seasonings. Serve hot for a satisfying and portable breakfast option that you can enjoy on the go.

4. **Egg Wrap**: To make an egg wrap, scramble eggs with your choice of vegetables, cheese, and cooked protein, then spoon the mixture onto a whole grain tortilla. Roll up the

tortilla and enjoy hot or cold for a quick and nutritious breakfast option that's perfect for busy mornings.

5. **Egg Salad**: To make egg salad, hard boil eggs and chop them into small pieces. Mix with Greek yogurt or mayonnaise, diced vegetables, herbs, and seasonings, then serve on whole grain bread or crackers for a satisfying and protein-rich breakfast option that you can enjoy at home or on the go.

By incorporating these simple egg recipes into your morning routine, you can enjoy a quick and satisfying breakfast that provides the energy and nutrients you need to start your day off right, even when time is short. Whether you prefer scrambled eggs, fried eggs, egg sandwiches, or egg wraps, there's a delicious and nutritious option to suit every taste preference and dietary need.

CHAPTER FOUR

Speedy Lunches for Busy Days

Lunchtime can often feel like a rushed affair, especially on busy days when time is of the essence. This subchapter is dedicated to providing quick and satisfying lunch ideas that can be prepared in a flash, ensuring that you can refuel and recharge without sacrificing precious time.

Fast and Filling Salad Recipes

Salads are a go-to option for quick and nutritious lunches, offering a perfect balance of fresh ingredients, vibrant flavors, and satisfying textures. This section showcases a variety of fast and filling salad recipes that are sure to keep you fueled and energized throughout the day.

1. **Mediterranean Chickpea Salad**: Combine chickpeas, cherry tomatoes, cucumber, red onion, olives, and feta cheese in a bowl. Dress with olive oil, lemon juice, garlic, and oregano for a refreshing and protein-packed salad that comes together in minutes.

2. **Asian Quinoa Salad**: Toss cooked quinoa with shredded carrots, edamame, red cabbage, bell peppers, and green onions. Drizzle with a sesame ginger dressing and top with sliced almonds and sesame seeds for a flavorful and nutrient-rich salad that's perfect for lunch on the go.

3. **Grilled Chicken Caesar Salad**: Top crisp romaine lettuce with grilled chicken breast, cherry tomatoes, parmesan cheese, and croutons. Drizzle with creamy Caesar dressing and toss to coat for a classic and satisfying salad that's ready in no time.

4. **Greek Orzo Salad**: Cook orzo pasta according to package instructions and toss with diced cucumber, cherry tomatoes, Kalamata olives, red onion, and feta cheese. Dress with olive oil, lemon juice, garlic, and fresh herbs for a refreshing and Mediterranean-inspired salad that's perfect for a quick lunch.

5. **Tuna Niçoise Salad**: Arrange mixed greens on a plate and top with canned tuna, boiled potatoes, blanched green beans, cherry tomatoes, hard-boiled eggs, and olives. Drizzle with a Dijon vinaigrette and garnish with fresh herbs for a hearty and satisfying salad that's both nutritious and delicious.

By incorporating these fast and filling salad recipes into your lunchtime repertoire, you can enjoy a nutritious and satisfying meal in no time, even on the busiest of days.

Sandwiches, Wraps, and Soup Ideas

Sandwiches, wraps, and soups are classic lunchtime staples that are perfect for busy days when time is short and hunger is looming. This section explores a variety of quick and convenient ideas for sandwiches, wraps, and soups that are sure to hit the spot.

1. **Turkey and Avocado Wrap**: Spread a whole grain tortilla with mashed avocado and layer with sliced turkey breast, lettuce, tomato, and cucumber. Roll up the wrap and enjoy a satisfying and protein-rich lunch that's perfect for eating on the go.

2. **Caprese Panini**: Layer sliced fresh mozzarella, tomato, and basil leaves on whole grain bread. Drizzle with balsamic glaze and grill in a panini press or skillet until the cheese is melted and the bread is golden brown. Serve hot for a delicious and gourmet-inspired lunch option.

3. **Vegetable and Bean Soup**: Sauté diced onion, carrots, celery, and garlic in olive oil until softened. Add vegetable broth, canned beans, diced tomatoes, and your choice of herbs and spices. Simmer until the vegetables are tender and the flavors are melded together, then serve hot for a comforting and nourishing lunch that's ready in minutes.

4. **Egg Salad Sandwich**: Mix chopped hard-boiled eggs with Greek yogurt or mayonnaise, diced celery, green onions, and Dijon mustard. Spread the egg salad onto whole grain bread and top with lettuce and tomato for a classic and satisfying sandwich that's perfect for a quick and easy lunch.

5. **Chicken and Vegetable Stir-Fry Wrap**: Sauté diced chicken breast with bell peppers, broccoli, and snap peas in a skillet until cooked through. Season with soy sauce, ginger, and garlic, then spoon the stir-fry onto a whole grain tortilla and roll up for a flavorful and protein-packed lunch option that's perfect for busy days.

Whether you prefer a hearty sandwich, a fresh wrap, or a comforting bowl of soup, these quick and convenient lunch ideas are sure to satisfy your hunger and keep you fueled throughout the day.

Lunches You Can Prep in 15 Minutes or Less

Prepping lunches ahead of time is a great way to save time and ensure that you have a nutritious meal ready to go when hunger strikes. This section highlights a variety of lunches that can be prepped in 15 minutes or less, making it easy to stay on track with your healthy eating goals even on the busiest of days.

1. **Mason Jar Salads**: Layer chopped vegetables, leafy greens, protein, and dressing in a mason jar for a portable and customizable lunch option that can be prepped ahead of time. Simply grab and go when you're ready to eat for a fresh and nutritious meal on the run.

2. **Cold Pasta Salad**: Toss cooked pasta with chopped vegetables, beans, cheese, and your choice of dressing for a simple and satisfying lunch option that can be enjoyed cold

or at room temperature. Pack individual portions in containers for easy grab-and-go lunches throughout the week.

3. **DIY Bento Box**: Fill a divided container with a variety of healthy and portable snacks, such as sliced vegetables, fruit, cheese, crackers, nuts, and hummus, for a fun and customizable lunch option that's perfect for on-the-go eating.

4. **Protein-Packed Snack Plate**: Arrange sliced hard-boiled eggs, cheese cubes, whole grain crackers, sliced vegetables, and hummus on a plate for a quick and easy lunch option that's packed with protein, fiber, and essential nutrients. Enjoy as is or pair with a piece of fruit for added sweetness and satisfaction.

5. **Leftover Stir-Fry**: Repurpose leftover stir-fry or cooked vegetables into a quick and satisfying lunch by reheating them in a skillet and serving over cooked rice or quinoa. Top with a fried egg or sliced avocado for added protein and flavor, then enjoy a delicious and nutritious meal that's ready in minutes.

By prepping lunches ahead of time and keeping quick and convenient options on hand, you can ensure that you always have a nutritious meal ready to go when hunger strikes, even on the busiest of days. Whether you prefer a salad, sandwich, wrap, soup, or snack plate, there's a quick and satisfying lunch option to suit every taste preference and dietary need.

CHAPTER FIVE

Dinner in a Flash: 15-Minute Entrees

Dinner is often the meal that requires the most time and effort, but it doesn't have to be that way. This subchapter is dedicated to showcasing a variety of entrees that can be prepared in just 15 minutes, allowing you to enjoy a delicious and satisfying dinner without spending hours in the kitchen.

Quick One-Pot Meals for Dinner

One-pot meals are a lifesaver on busy weeknights, offering a convenient and efficient way to prepare dinner without creating a mountain of dishes to clean up afterward. This section highlights a variety of quick one-pot meals that are perfect for dinner in a flash.

1. **Pasta Primavera**: Cook pasta according to package instructions, adding vegetables like bell peppers, zucchini, cherry tomatoes, and spinach to the pot during the last few minutes of cooking. Drain the pasta and vegetables, then toss with olive oil, garlic, herbs, and grated parmesan cheese for a quick and flavorful dinner option that's ready in minutes.

2. **One-Pot Chicken and Rice**: Sauté diced chicken breast in a skillet until cooked through, then add rice, chicken broth, diced vegetables, and seasonings to the pot. Cover and

simmer until the rice is tender and the liquid is absorbed, then fluff with a fork and serve hot for a comforting and satisfying dinner option that requires minimal effort.

3. **Vegetarian Chili**: Sauté diced onion, bell peppers, and garlic in a large pot until softened, then add canned beans, diced tomatoes, vegetable broth, and spices. Simmer for a few minutes until heated through, then serve hot with toppings like avocado, cheese, and cilantro for a hearty and nutritious dinner option that's perfect for chilly evenings.

4. **Shrimp and Vegetable Stir-Fry**: Sauté shrimp, diced vegetables, and garlic in a skillet until the shrimp is pink and the vegetables are tender-crisp. Season with soy sauce, ginger, and sesame oil, then serve hot over cooked rice or noodles for a quick and flavorful dinner option that's ready in minutes.

5. **Quinoa and Black Bean Skillet**: Cook quinoa according to package instructions, then sauté diced onion, bell peppers, and garlic in a skillet until softened. Add cooked quinoa, canned black beans, diced tomatoes, and spices to the skillet, then simmer until heated through. Serve hot with toppings like avocado, Greek yogurt, and fresh herbs for a protein-packed and satisfying dinner option that's perfect for busy weeknights.

By incorporating these quick one-pot meals into your dinner rotation, you can enjoy a delicious and satisfying meal with minimal time and effort, leaving you more time to relax and unwind after a long day.

Sheet Pan Dinners for Effortless Cooking

Sheet pan dinners are a game-changer when it comes to quick and effortless cooking, offering a simple and efficient way to prepare a complete meal with minimal fuss and cleanup. This section explores a variety of sheet pan dinner ideas that are perfect for busy evenings when time is short.

1. **Baked Salmon and Vegetables**: Place salmon fillets on a sheet pan and surround them with your favorite vegetables, such as asparagus, broccoli, and cherry tomatoes. Drizzle everything with olive oil, lemon juice, and herbs, then bake in the oven until the salmon is cooked through and the vegetables are tender for a nutritious and flavorful dinner option that's ready in minutes.

2. **Chicken Fajita Sheet Pan Dinner**: Arrange sliced chicken breast, bell peppers, onions, and spices on a sheet pan and toss everything together until evenly coated. Roast in the oven until the chicken is cooked through and the vegetables are tender, then serve hot with tortillas, salsa, and toppings like avocado and cheese for a quick and satisfying dinner option that's perfect for busy nights.

3. **Roasted Sausage and Potatoes**: Slice smoked sausage and potatoes and place them on a sheet pan along with diced bell peppers and onions. Drizzle with olive oil, garlic, and herbs, then roast in the oven until the sausage is browned and the potatoes are tender for a hearty and comforting dinner option that's ready in minutes.

4. **Vegetable and Chickpea Sheet Pan Curry**: Toss diced vegetables, chickpeas, and curry paste together on a sheet pan until evenly coated. Roast in the oven until the vegetables are tender and the chickpeas are crispy, then serve hot over cooked rice or quinoa for a flavorful and nutritious dinner option that's perfect for busy evenings.

5. **Sausage and Vegetable Sheet Pan Hash**: Slice smoked sausage and potatoes and place them on a sheet pan along with diced vegetables like bell peppers, onions, and zucchini. Drizzle with olive oil, garlic, and herbs, then roast in the oven until everything is tender and golden brown for a hearty and satisfying dinner option that's ready in minutes.

Sheet pan dinners are not only quick and convenient, but they also offer endless possibilities for customization and creativity, making them a versatile and practical option for busy weeknights.

Stir-Fries and Skillet Dishes Ready in Minutes

Stir-fries and skillet dishes are perfect for quick and flavorful dinners, offering a simple and efficient way to prepare a complete meal in just minutes. This section showcases a variety of stir-fry and skillet dish ideas that are perfect for busy evenings when time is short.

1. **Beef and Broccoli Stir-Fry**: Sauté sliced beef, broccoli florets, and garlic in a skillet until the beef is browned and the broccoli is tender-crisp. Season with soy sauce, ginger, and sesame oil, then serve hot over cooked rice or noodles for a quick and satisfying dinner option that's ready in minutes.

2. **Vegetable and Tofu Stir-Fry**: Sauté diced tofu, bell peppers, snap peas, and carrots in a skillet until the tofu is golden brown and the vegetables are tender-crisp. Season with soy sauce, garlic, and ginger, then serve hot over cooked rice or noodles for a protein-packed and nutritious dinner option that's perfect for busy nights.

3. **Shrimp and Vegetable Skillet**: Sauté shrimp, diced vegetables, and garlic in a skillet until the shrimp is pink and the vegetables are tender-crisp. Season with lemon juice, herbs, and spices, then serve hot over cooked quinoa or couscous for a quick and flavorful dinner option that's ready in minutes.

4. **Teriyaki Chicken and Vegetable Stir-Fry**: Sauté sliced chicken breast, bell peppers, onions, and snap peas in a skillet until the chicken is cooked through and the vegetables are tender-crisp. Drizzle with teriyaki sauce and toss to coat,

then serve hot over cooked rice or noodles for a quick and satisfying dinner option that's perfect for busy evenings.

5. **Pork and Vegetable Stir-Fry**: Sauté sliced pork tenderloin, bell peppers, broccoli, and garlic in a skillet until the pork is browned and the vegetables are tender-crisp. Season with soy sauce, ginger, and sesame oil, then serve hot over cooked rice or noodles for a flavorful and satisfying dinner option that's ready in minutes.

Stir-fries and skillet dishes are not only quick and easy to prepare, but they also offer endless possibilities for customization and creativity, making them a versatile and practical option for busy weeknights. Whether you prefer beef and broccoli stir-fry, vegetable and tofu stir-fry, or shrimp and vegetable skillet, there's a quick and flavorful option to suit every taste preference and dietary need.

CHAPTER SIX

Snacks to Satisfy in Seconds

Snacking plays a crucial role in maintaining energy levels and preventing hunger between meals. This subchapter is dedicated to providing a variety of quick and satisfying snack ideas that can be enjoyed in seconds, ensuring that you can refuel and stay energized throughout the day.

Healthy Snacks to Curb Hunger Between Meals

Healthy snacks are essential for keeping hunger at bay and preventing overeating during mealtime. This section offers a variety of nutritious snack ideas that are perfect for curbing hunger between meals.

1. **Greek Yogurt with Berries**: Greek yogurt is rich in protein and calcium, making it a satisfying snack option that can help keep you feeling full between meals. Top with fresh berries for added sweetness and fiber, creating a delicious and nutritious snack that's perfect for any time of day.

2. **Apple Slices with Nut Butter**: Apples are a convenient and portable snack option that's packed with fiber and vitamins. Pair them with your favorite nut butter, such as almond or peanut butter, for a satisfying combination of sweet and savory flavors that will keep you satisfied until your next meal.

3. **Raw Vegetables with Hummus**: Raw vegetables, such as carrots, celery, cucumber, and bell peppers, are low in calories and high in fiber, making them an excellent snack choice for curbing hunger between meals. Dip them in hummus for added flavor and protein, creating a crunchy and satisfying snack that's perfect for munching on throughout the day.

4. **Mixed Nuts and Dried Fruit**: A handful of mixed nuts and dried fruit is a convenient and satisfying snack option that's perfect for curbing hunger on the go. Choose unsalted nuts and opt for dried fruit without added sugars for a nutritious and delicious snack that provides a combination of protein, healthy fats, and carbohydrates.

5. **Whole Grain Crackers with Cheese**: Whole grain crackers are a convenient and satisfying snack option that's perfect for curbing hunger between meals. Pair them with your favorite cheese for added protein and flavor, creating a delicious and nutritious snack that's perfect for any time of day.

By incorporating these healthy snacks into your daily routine, you can keep hunger at bay and ensure that you have the energy you need to tackle whatever the day throws your way.

Portable Snacks for On-the-Go Convenience

On-the-go snacks are essential for busy days when you need a quick and convenient option to keep you fueled and energized.

This section highlights a variety of portable snack ideas that are perfect for enjoying on the go.

1. **Trail Mix**: Trail mix is a convenient and portable snack option that's perfect for on-the-go convenience. Mix together nuts, dried fruit, and dark chocolate chips for a satisfying combination of sweet and savory flavors that's perfect for munching on throughout the day.

2. **Granola Bars**: Granola bars are a convenient and portable snack option that's perfect for on-the-go convenience. Choose options that are low in added sugars and high in fiber and protein for a nutritious and satisfying snack that will keep you fueled and energized throughout the day.

3. **String Cheese**: String cheese is a convenient and portable snack option that's perfect for on-the-go convenience. Pair it with whole grain crackers or fresh fruit for added flavor and nutrition, creating a delicious and satisfying snack that's perfect for any time of day.

4. **Energy Bites**: Energy bites are a convenient and portable snack option that's perfect for on-the-go convenience. Made with ingredients like oats, nut butter, and honey, they're packed with protein, fiber, and healthy fats, making them a nutritious and delicious snack that will keep you fueled and energized throughout the day.

5. **Yogurt Parfait Cups**: Yogurt parfait cups are a convenient and portable snack option that's perfect for on-the-go convenience. Layer Greek yogurt with fresh fruit and granola in a small container for a satisfying combination of protein, fiber, and vitamins that's perfect for enjoying on the go.

By keeping these portable snacks on hand, you can ensure that you always have a quick and convenient option to keep you fueled and energized throughout the day, no matter how busy your schedule may be.

Quick and Easy Snack Recipes for Anytime

Sometimes, the best snacks are the ones you make yourself. This section offers a variety of quick and easy snack recipes that are perfect for enjoying anytime, whether you're craving something sweet, savory, or satisfying.

1. **Homemade Trail Mix**: Mix together your favorite nuts, dried fruit, seeds, and dark chocolate chips for a customized trail mix that's perfect for snacking on throughout the day. Store in individual portion-sized bags or containers for easy grab-and-go convenience.

2. **No-Bake Energy Bars**: Combine oats, nut butter, honey, and your favorite mix-ins like nuts, seeds, and dried fruit in a bowl. Press the mixture into a baking dish and refrigerate until firm, then cut into bars for a quick and satisfying snack option that's perfect for anytime.

3. **Vegetable Sushi Rolls**: Spread cooked sushi rice onto a sheet of nori and top with thinly sliced vegetables like cucumber, avocado, and bell peppers. Roll up the nori tightly and slice into bite-sized pieces for a refreshing and nutritious snack option that's perfect for enjoying anytime.

4. **Fruit and Yogurt Popsicles**: Blend together your favorite fruits with Greek yogurt and a touch of honey until smooth. Pour the mixture into popsicle molds and freeze until solid, then enjoy a refreshing and satisfying snack that's perfect for cooling off on hot days.

5. **Caprese Skewers**: Thread cherry tomatoes, fresh mozzarella balls, and basil leaves onto skewers for a quick and easy snack option that's perfect for anytime. Drizzle with balsamic glaze and olive oil for added flavor and enjoy a delicious and satisfying snack that's perfect for any occasion.

By making your own quick and easy snack recipes at home, you can ensure that you always have a nutritious and satisfying option to enjoy anytime, whether you're at home, at work, or on the go. Whether you prefer homemade trail mix, no-bake energy bars, vegetable sushi rolls, fruit and yogurt popsicles, or Caprese skewers, there's a quick and easy snack recipe to suit every taste preference and dietary need.

CHAPTER SEVEN

Speedy Sides to Complete Your Meals

Completing a meal with the perfect side dish can elevate the dining experience. This subchapter delves into a variety of quick and easy side dish ideas that can complement any main course, ensuring that your meals are balanced and satisfying.

Fast Vegetable Side Dishes

Vegetables are an essential component of a balanced meal, providing essential nutrients and vibrant flavors. This section offers a range of vegetable side dish ideas that are quick to prepare and bursting with freshness.

1. **Sautéed Garlic Green Beans**: Heat olive oil in a skillet over medium heat and add trimmed green beans and minced garlic. Sauté until the green beans are tender-crisp and lightly browned, then season with salt and pepper to taste. Garnish with freshly chopped parsley for a simple yet flavorful vegetable side dish that pairs well with a variety of main courses.

2. **Roasted Parmesan Brussels Sprouts**: Toss halved Brussels sprouts with olive oil, grated Parmesan cheese, salt, and pepper on a baking sheet. Roast in the oven at 400°F (200°C) for 15-20 minutes until the Brussels sprouts are caramelized and tender. Serve hot for a delicious and nutritious vegetable side dish that's sure to please even the pickiest eaters.

3. **Stir-Fried Sesame Broccoli**: Heat sesame oil in a wok or skillet over high heat and add broccoli florets. Stir-fry until the broccoli is crisp-tender, then add soy sauce, minced garlic, and sesame seeds. Continue to stir-fry for another minute until the broccoli is coated in the sauce and heated through. Serve hot for a quick and flavorful vegetable side dish that's perfect for Asian-inspired meals.

4. **Honey Glazed Carrots**: Steam or boil baby carrots until tender, then drain and return them to the pot. Add butter, honey, and a pinch of cinnamon to the carrots and toss until evenly coated. Cook for another minute until the honey glaze thickens slightly, then serve hot for a sweet and savory vegetable side dish that's perfect for family dinners or special occasions.

5. **Grilled Asparagus with Lemon Zest**: Preheat a grill or grill pan over medium-high heat and brush trimmed asparagus spears with olive oil. Grill the asparagus for 2-3 minutes per side until lightly charred and tender. Remove from the grill and sprinkle with lemon zest and a squeeze of fresh lemon juice before serving. Enjoy hot for a simple yet elegant vegetable side dish that pairs well with grilled meats and seafood.

By incorporating these fast vegetable side dishes into your meal rotation, you can add a burst of color, flavor, and nutrition to any plate with minimal effort.

Quick and Healthy Grain Side Dishes

Grains are a versatile and nutritious addition to any meal, providing essential carbohydrates and fiber. This section explores a variety of quick and healthy grain side dishes that can complement a wide range of main courses.

1. **Quinoa Pilaf with Mixed Herbs**: Rinse quinoa under cold water, then cook according to package instructions in vegetable or chicken broth for added flavor. Once cooked, fluff the quinoa with a fork and stir in a mixture of freshly chopped herbs such as parsley, cilantro, and dill. Season with salt and pepper to taste and serve hot for a light and flavorful grain side dish that's perfect for pairing with grilled or roasted meats.

2. **Brown Rice Stir-Fry with Vegetables**: Cook brown rice according to package instructions, then set aside. Heat sesame oil in a wok or skillet over high heat and add diced vegetables such as bell peppers, carrots, and snap peas. Stir-fry until the vegetables are crisp-tender, then add the cooked brown rice and soy sauce. Continue to stir-fry until everything is heated through and well combined. Serve hot

for a quick and healthy grain side dish that's perfect for Asian-inspired meals.

3. **Millet Salad with Lemon Vinaigrette**: Cook millet according to package instructions, then let it cool to room temperature. In a large bowl, toss the cooked millet with diced cucumber, cherry tomatoes, red onion, and crumbled feta cheese. Drizzle with a homemade lemon vinaigrette made with olive oil, lemon juice, garlic, and Dijon mustard. Toss until everything is well coated and serve chilled for a refreshing and nutritious grain side dish that's perfect for summer barbecues and picnics.

4. **Couscous with Mediterranean Vegetables**: Prepare couscous according to package instructions, then set aside. In a large skillet, sauté diced eggplant, zucchini, bell peppers, and cherry tomatoes in olive oil until tender. Season with dried oregano, basil, and a pinch of red pepper flakes for added flavor. Serve the sautéed vegetables over the cooked couscous and garnish with crumbled feta cheese and chopped fresh parsley. Enjoy hot for a flavorful and satisfying grain side dish that's perfect for vegetarian meals or as a complement to grilled meats.

5. **Barley and Mushroom Risotto**: Cook pearl barley according to package instructions, then set aside. In a large skillet, sauté sliced mushrooms in butter until golden brown and

tender. Add minced garlic and thyme to the skillet and cook for another minute until fragrant. Stir in the cooked barley and vegetable broth, then simmer until the broth is absorbed and the barley is creamy and tender. Serve hot with grated Parmesan cheese and chopped parsley for a comforting and hearty grain side dish that's perfect for cozy dinners at home.

By incorporating these quick and healthy grain side dishes into your meal repertoire, you can add texture, flavor, and nutritional value to any plate with minimal effort.

Low-Carb Alternatives to Traditional Sides

For those following a low-carb or ketogenic diet, traditional grain-based side dishes may not be suitable. This section offers a variety of low-carb alternatives to traditional sides that are satisfying, flavorful, and easy to prepare.

1. **Cauliflower Rice Pilaf**: Grate cauliflower florets using a box grater or pulse them in a food processor until they resemble rice grains. Sauté the cauliflower rice in olive oil with diced onion, minced garlic, and your choice of herbs and spices until tender. Stir in toasted nuts, dried fruit, and chopped fresh herbs for added flavor and texture. Serve hot for a low-carb alternative to traditional rice pilaf that's perfect for pairing with grilled or roasted meats.

2. **Zucchini Noodles with Pesto**: Use a spiralizer to create long strands of zucchini noodles, then sauté them in olive oil until tender. Toss the cooked zucchini noodles with homemade or store-bought pesto until evenly coated. Serve hot or cold for a flavorful and low-carb alternative to traditional pasta dishes that's perfect for summer meals or as a light and refreshing side dish.

3. **Spaghetti Squash Alfredo**: Cut spaghetti squash in half lengthwise and remove the seeds. Place the squash halves cut-side down on a baking sheet and roast in the oven at 400°F (200°C) for 40-45 minutes until tender. Use a fork to scrape the flesh of the squash into long strands, then toss with homemade or store-bought Alfredo sauce until evenly coated. Serve hot for a creamy and indulgent low-carb alternative to traditional pasta dishes that's perfect for satisfying comfort food cravings.

4. **Broccoli Cauliflower Mash**: Steam or boil equal parts broccoli florets and cauliflower florets until tender, then drain well. Transfer the cooked broccoli and cauliflower to a food processor and pulse until smooth. Stir in butter, cream cheese, minced garlic, and grated Parmesan cheese until well combined. Season with salt and pepper to taste and serve hot for a creamy and flavorful low-carb alternative to

traditional mashed potatoes that's perfect for serving alongside grilled meats or roasted vegetables.

5. **Green Bean Fries**: Trim and blanch fresh green beans in boiling water for 2-3 minutes until crisp-tender, then drain well. Toss the blanched green beans with olive oil, grated Parmesan cheese, and your choice of herbs and spices until evenly coated. Arrange the seasoned green beans in a single layer on a baking sheet and roast in the oven at 425°F (220°C) for 15-20 minutes until golden brown and crispy. Serve hot for a crunchy and satisfying low-carb alternative to traditional french fries that's perfect for snacking or serving as a side dish.

By incorporating these low-carb alternatives to traditional sides into your meal planning, you can enjoy all the flavors and textures of your favorite dishes without the added carbs, making it easier to stick to your dietary goals and enjoy delicious and satisfying meals. Whether you prefer cauliflower rice pilaf, zucchini noodles with pesto, spaghetti squash Alfredo, broccoli cauliflower mash, or green bean fries, there's a low-carb alternative to traditional sides to suit every taste preference and dietary need.

CHAPTER EIGHT

Desserts in the Blink of an Eye

Desserts are the perfect way to cap off a delicious meal, but they don't have to be time-consuming to prepare. This subchapter explores a variety of quick and easy dessert ideas that can be whipped up in a flash, ensuring that you can satisfy your sweet tooth with minimal effort.

Sweet Treats for Quick Indulgence

Sometimes, you just need a little something sweet to satisfy your cravings. This section offers a range of sweet treats that can be prepared in minutes, allowing you to indulge your sweet tooth without spending hours in the kitchen.

1. **Microwave Mug Cakes**: Combine flour, sugar, cocoa powder, baking powder, milk, and oil in a microwave-safe mug. Stir until well combined, then microwave on high for 1-2 minutes until the cake is set. Top with whipped cream or ice cream for a quick and indulgent dessert that's perfect for satisfying sudden cravings.

2. **No-Bake Cookies**: Combine peanut butter, oats, honey, and cocoa powder in a bowl until well combined. Drop spoonfuls of the mixture onto a parchment-lined baking sheet and refrigerate until firm. Enjoy these sweet and chewy cookies

straight from the fridge for a quick and satisfying treat that requires no baking.

3. **Fruit and Yogurt Parfaits**: Layer Greek yogurt with fresh fruit, granola, and a drizzle of honey in a glass or bowl for a quick and healthy dessert option that's perfect for any time of day. Customize your parfait with your favorite fruits and toppings for endless flavor possibilities.

4. **Frozen Banana Bites**: Slice bananas into rounds and spread peanut butter or Nutella on half of the slices. Top with the remaining banana slices to create sandwiches, then dip each banana sandwich into melted chocolate and freeze until firm. Enjoy these creamy and indulgent treats straight from the freezer for a quick and satisfying dessert option.

5. **Quick Berry Crumbles**: Toss fresh or frozen berries with a little sugar and cornstarch, then divide the mixture into individual ramekins. Top with a mixture of oats, flour, brown sugar, and butter, then bake in the oven at 375°F (190°C) for 15-20 minutes until golden brown and bubbly. Serve hot with a scoop of vanilla ice cream for a comforting and delicious dessert that's ready in no time.

By incorporating these sweet treats into your dessert repertoire, you can satisfy your cravings for something sweet without spending hours in the kitchen.

Fruit-Based Desserts for Natural Sweetness

Fruit is nature's candy, offering natural sweetness and vibrant flavors that are perfect for satisfying your sweet tooth. This section explores a variety of fruit-based dessert ideas that are quick and easy to prepare.

1. **Grilled Fruit Skewers**: Thread chunks of pineapple, mango, banana, and strawberries onto skewers and grill for a few minutes on each side until lightly charred and caramelized. Serve these warm and juicy fruit skewers with a drizzle of honey or a scoop of vanilla ice cream for a delicious and refreshing dessert option that's perfect for summer barbecues and gatherings.

2. **Frozen Yogurt Bark**: Spread Greek yogurt onto a parchment-lined baking sheet and top with a mixture of fresh fruit, nuts, and seeds. Freeze until firm, then break into pieces and enjoy this creamy and refreshing dessert straight from the freezer for a quick and satisfying treat that's perfect for hot summer days.

3. **Fruit Salad with Honey Lime Dressing**: Toss together a variety of fresh fruit such as strawberries, blueberries, kiwi, pineapple, and grapes in a large bowl. Drizzle with a mixture of honey, lime juice, and mint leaves for a sweet and tangy dressing that enhances the natural flavors of the fruit. Serve

chilled for a refreshing and nutritious dessert option that's perfect for any occasion.

4. **Baked Apples with Cinnamon**: Core apples and place them in a baking dish. Fill each apple cavity with a mixture of brown sugar, cinnamon, and butter, then bake in the oven at 375°F (190°C) for 20-25 minutes until the apples are tender and caramelized. Serve hot with a dollop of whipped cream or a scoop of vanilla ice cream for a comforting and satisfying dessert option that's perfect for fall and winter.

5. **Chocolate-Dipped Strawberries**: Dip fresh strawberries into melted chocolate and place them on a parchment-lined baking sheet. Refrigerate until the chocolate is set, then serve these elegant and indulgent treats as a quick and easy dessert option for special occasions or as a sweet ending to any meal.

By incorporating these fruit-based desserts into your meal planning, you can enjoy the natural sweetness and vibrant flavors of fresh fruit in a variety of delicious and satisfying ways.

Simple Sugar-Free Dessert Recipes

For those looking to reduce their sugar intake, there are plenty of delicious dessert options that are naturally sweetened or sugar-free. This section offers a range of simple and satisfying dessert recipes that are free from refined sugars.

1. **Chia Seed Pudding**: Combine chia seeds, almond milk, and a touch of vanilla extract in a jar or bowl. Stir until well combined, then refrigerate for at least 4 hours or overnight until the mixture thickens and becomes pudding-like in texture. Serve chilled with fresh fruit and a sprinkle of cinnamon for a creamy and satisfying dessert option that's naturally sweetened and packed with nutrients.

2. **Coconut Flour Pancakes**: Combine coconut flour, eggs, almond milk, and a pinch of baking powder in a bowl until well combined. Cook spoonfuls of the batter in a skillet greased with coconut oil until golden brown and cooked through. Serve these fluffy and delicious pancakes with a drizzle of sugar-free maple syrup or a dollop of Greek yogurt for a quick and satisfying dessert option that's perfect for breakfast or brunch.

3. **Avocado Chocolate Mousse**: Blend ripe avocados, cocoa powder, almond milk, and a touch of honey or maple syrup in a blender or food processor until smooth and creamy. Divide the mousse into individual serving glasses and refrigerate for at least 1 hour until chilled and set. Serve with a dollop of whipped cream or a sprinkle of cocoa powder for a rich and indulgent dessert option that's naturally sweetened and packed with healthy fats.

4. **Sugar-Free Fruit Sorbet**: Blend frozen fruit such as berries, mango, or pineapple in a blender or food processor until smooth and creamy. Add a splash of lemon juice or coconut water to help the mixture blend smoothly, then transfer to a shallow dish and freeze for at least 4 hours or overnight until firm. Serve this refreshing and guilt-free sorbet as a quick and satisfying dessert option that's perfect for cooling off on hot summer days.

5. **Almond Flour Cookies**: Combine almond flour, eggs, coconut oil, and a touch of vanilla extract in a bowl until well combined. Fold in your choice of mix-ins such as dark chocolate chips, chopped nuts, or dried fruit. Drop spoonfuls of the dough onto a parchment-lined baking sheet and bake in the oven at 350°F (180°C) for 10-12 minutes until golden brown and cooked through. Enjoy these chewy and delicious cookies as a quick and satisfying dessert option that's free from refined sugars.

By incorporating these simple sugar-free dessert recipes into your meal planning, you can enjoy all the flavors and textures of your favorite desserts without the added sugars, making it easier to stick to your dietary goals and enjoy delicious and satisfying treats. Whether you prefer chia seed pudding, coconut flour pancakes, avocado chocolate mousse, sugar-free fruit sorbet, or almond flour cookies, there's a sugar-free dessert recipe to suit every taste preference and dietary need.

CHAPTER NINE

15-Minute Meals on the Go

Balancing a busy schedule with the need to eat well can be a challenge, but with the right recipes and strategies, it's possible to enjoy quick and nutritious meals even when you're on the go. This subchapter explores a variety of 15-minute meal ideas designed for busy individuals who need fast and convenient options that don't sacrifice flavor or nutrition.

Quick and Healthy Meals for Busy Days

When time is limited, it's essential to have a repertoire of quick and healthy meal ideas that can be prepared in a flash. This section offers a range of nutritious meal options that can be whipped up in just 15 minutes, ensuring that you can enjoy a satisfying and balanced meal even on the busiest of days.

1. **Turkey and Veggie Stir-Fry**: Heat olive oil in a skillet over high heat and add sliced turkey breast and diced vegetables such as bell peppers, broccoli, and snap peas. Stir-fry until the turkey is cooked through and the vegetables are crisp-tender, then season with soy sauce, garlic, and ginger. Serve hot over cooked rice or quinoa for a quick and flavorful meal that's packed with protein and fiber.

2. **Mediterranean Chickpea Salad**: In a large bowl, toss together canned chickpeas, diced cucumber, cherry

tomatoes, red onion, and crumbled feta cheese. Drizzle with olive oil, lemon juice, and a sprinkle of dried oregano, then season with salt and pepper to taste. Serve chilled for a refreshing and nutritious meal option that's perfect for lunch or dinner.

3. **Shrimp Tacos with Avocado Salsa**: Heat a skillet over medium-high heat and add shrimp seasoned with chili powder, cumin, and garlic powder. Cook for 2-3 minutes per side until pink and cooked through, then assemble the tacos with corn tortillas, shredded cabbage, and homemade avocado salsa made with diced avocado, tomatoes, onions, cilantro, and lime juice. Serve hot for a quick and satisfying meal that's bursting with flavor.

4. **Caprese Pasta Salad**: Cook pasta according to package instructions, then drain and rinse under cold water to cool. In a large bowl, toss the cooked pasta with halved cherry tomatoes, fresh mozzarella balls, chopped basil leaves, and a drizzle of balsamic glaze. Season with salt and pepper to taste and serve chilled for a simple yet delicious meal option that's perfect for picnics or packed lunches.

5. **Asian Beef Lettuce Wraps**: Sauté ground beef with diced onions, garlic, and ginger in a skillet until browned and cooked through. Stir in hoisin sauce, soy sauce, and sesame oil, then spoon the beef mixture onto large lettuce leaves.

Top with shredded carrots, sliced green onions, and chopped peanuts for added crunch and flavor. Serve immediately for a quick and satisfying meal that's perfect for busy weeknights.

By incorporating these quick and healthy meal ideas into your repertoire, you can ensure that you have nutritious options on hand that can be prepared in just 15 minutes, making it easier to eat well even when you're short on time.

Portable Lunches and Snacks for Work or School

When you're on the go, having portable lunch and snack options can help you stay fueled and energized throughout the day. This section offers a variety of convenient meal and snack ideas that are perfect for taking with you to work or school.

1. **Mason Jar Salads**: Layer salad ingredients such as greens, chopped vegetables, cooked grains, beans, and proteins in a mason jar, starting with the dressing on the bottom and ending with the lettuce on top. Seal the jar tightly and refrigerate until ready to eat, then shake to distribute the dressing and enjoy a fresh and flavorful salad on the go.

2. **Bento Box Lunches**: Pack a bento box with a variety of portable and nutritious foods such as sliced vegetables, cheese cubes, whole grain crackers, boiled eggs, and fresh fruit. Customize your bento box with your favorite foods and

flavors for a balanced and satisfying meal option that's perfect for taking with you wherever you go.

3. **Protein-Packed Snack Boxes**: Fill small containers or snack bags with protein-rich foods such as nuts, seeds, Greek yogurt, hard-boiled eggs, and sliced turkey or chicken breast. Keep these snack boxes on hand for quick and convenient energy boosts throughout the day, whether you're at work, school, or on the go.

4. **Homemade Energy Bars**: Make your own energy bars using ingredients like oats, nuts, seeds, dried fruit, and nut butter. Press the mixture into a baking dish and refrigerate until firm, then cut into bars or squares for a portable and nutritious snack option that's perfect for refueling on busy days.

5. **Veggie and Hummus Wraps**: Spread hummus onto a whole wheat tortilla and top with sliced vegetables such as cucumbers, bell peppers, carrots, and spinach leaves. Roll up the tortilla tightly and slice into pinwheels for a convenient and nutritious snack or light meal option that's perfect for taking with you on the go.

By preparing these portable lunches and snacks ahead of time, you can ensure that you always have convenient options on hand to keep you fueled and energized throughout the day, no matter how busy your schedule may be.

Tips for Eating Well When Pressed for Time

In addition to having quick and convenient meal and snack options on hand, there are several strategies you can use to ensure that you're able to eat well even when you're pressed for time. This section offers a variety of tips and tricks for maintaining a healthy diet on busy days.

1. **Plan Ahead**: Take a few minutes at the beginning of each week to plan out your meals and snacks for the upcoming days. This will help you make healthier choices and avoid the temptation to grab fast food or convenience meals when you're short on time.

2. **Prep Ingredients in Advance**: Spend some time prepping ingredients such as chopped vegetables, cooked grains, and grilled proteins at the beginning of the week. Store them in separate containers in the fridge so that you can easily assemble meals and snacks throughout the week without having to spend time chopping and cooking every day.

3. **Use Time-Saving Kitchen Tools**: Invest in time-saving kitchen tools such as a slow cooker, pressure cooker, or immersion blender to help you prepare meals more quickly and efficiently. These tools can help you whip up nutritious meals in a fraction of the time it would take to cook them on the stove or in the oven.

4. **Keep Healthy Staples on Hand**: Stock your pantry, fridge, and freezer with healthy staples such as canned beans, whole grains, frozen vegetables, and lean proteins. Having these ingredients on hand will make it easier to throw together quick and nutritious meals without having to make a trip to the grocery store.

5. **Practice Mindful Eating**: Take the time to sit down and savor your meals, even when you're on the go. Eating mindfully can help you enjoy your food more fully and prevent overeating, leading to better digestion and satisfaction.

By incorporating these tips into your daily routine, you can ensure that you're able to eat well even when you're pressed for time, making it easier to maintain a healthy diet and lifestyle no matter how busy your schedule may be.

CHAPTER TEN

Mastering Quick Diabetic Cooking Habits

Efficient and quick cooking habits are essential for managing diabetes without sacrificing flavor or nutrition. This subchapter explores strategies and tips to master quick diabetic cooking habits, ensuring that you can prepare delicious and balanced meals in minimal time.

Strategies for Efficient Meal Planning

Meal planning is the cornerstone of efficient cooking, especially when managing diabetes. This section offers strategies to streamline meal planning and ensure that you have nutritious meals ready to go in a pinch.

1. **Plan Weekly Menus**: Set aside time each week to plan your meals for the upcoming days. Consider your schedule, dietary needs, and preferences when creating your menu, and aim for a balance of protein, carbohydrates, and healthy fats in each meal.

2. **Batch Cooking**: Cook large batches of staple foods such as grains, beans, and proteins on your designated meal prep day. Portion them out into containers and store them in the fridge or freezer for easy access throughout the week. This allows you to assemble meals quickly without having to start from scratch each time.

3. **Prep Ingredients in Advance**: Chop vegetables, marinate proteins, and portion out ingredients ahead of time to streamline the cooking process. Store prepped ingredients in airtight containers or resealable bags in the fridge so that they're ready to go when you need them.

4. **Use Time-Saving Kitchen Tools**: Invest in kitchen tools that can help you save time and effort, such as a slow cooker, pressure cooker, or food processor. These tools can help you cook meals more quickly and efficiently, allowing you to spend less time in the kitchen.

5. **Keep a Well-Stocked Pantry**: Stock your pantry with essential ingredients such as canned beans, diced tomatoes, whole grains, and low-sodium broths. Having these staples on hand allows you to throw together quick and nutritious meals without having to make a trip to the store.

By implementing these meal planning strategies, you can streamline your cooking process and ensure that you always have healthy and delicious meals on hand, even when time is tight.

Tips for Speedy Kitchen Clean-Up

Efficient kitchen clean-up is just as important as efficient meal preparation, especially when cooking quick diabetic meals. This section offers tips to speed up the kitchen clean-up process and maintain a tidy cooking environment.

1. **Clean As You Go**: Wash dishes, utensils, and cutting boards as you cook to prevent clutter and make clean-up easier once the meal is finished. This helps to minimize the amount of time spent cleaning up after cooking and ensures that your kitchen stays organized throughout the process.

2. **Use One-Pot Meals**: Opt for one-pot meals whenever possible to minimize the number of dishes that need to be washed. Not only does this reduce clean-up time, but it also simplifies the cooking process and allows flavors to meld together for delicious results.

3. **Line Baking Sheets and Pans**: Line baking sheets and pans with parchment paper or aluminum foil before cooking to make clean-up a breeze. Simply remove the liner after cooking, and you'll be left with a clean pan that requires minimal scrubbing.

4. **Delegate Tasks**: If you have family members or roommates, enlist their help with kitchen clean-up to speed up the process. Assign specific tasks such as washing dishes, wiping down countertops, or putting away leftovers to divide and conquer the clean-up process.

5. **Invest in Quality Cleaning Supplies**: Stock your kitchen with quality cleaning supplies such as dish soap, sponges, and scrub brushes to make clean-up easier and more efficient.

Having the right tools on hand can help you tackle tough messes quickly and effectively.

By incorporating these tips into your kitchen routine, you can streamline the clean-up process and ensure that your cooking environment stays tidy and organized, allowing you to focus on enjoying your delicious diabetic meals.

Making 15-Minute Meals a Sustainable Lifestyle

Creating a sustainable lifestyle around 15-minute meals requires commitment and consistency. This section offers tips to make quick diabetic cooking habits a permanent part of your routine.

1. **Set Realistic Expectations**: Understand that not every meal needs to be prepared in 15 minutes flat. Aim to incorporate quick meals into your routine a few times a week and allow yourself flexibility for longer cooking sessions when time permits.

2. **Experiment with Recipes**: Keep things interesting by trying out new recipes and flavors. Experiment with different ingredients, cooking techniques, and cuisines to keep your meals varied and exciting, even when time is limited.

3. **Listen to Your Body**: Pay attention to how different foods affect your blood sugar levels and energy levels throughout the day. Adjust your meals and portion sizes accordingly to

ensure that you're maintaining stable blood sugar levels while still enjoying delicious and satisfying meals.

4. **Make It a Habit**: Consistency is key when it comes to creating sustainable habits. Make quick diabetic cooking a regular part of your routine by setting aside dedicated time for meal planning, grocery shopping, and cooking each week.

5. **Celebrate Your Successes**: Acknowledge and celebrate your achievements along the way. Whether you successfully whip up a 15-minute meal on a busy weeknight or master a new cooking technique, take pride in your accomplishments and use them as motivation to keep pushing forward on your journey to better health.

By following these tips, you can create a sustainable lifestyle centered around quick diabetic cooking habits, ensuring that you're able to enjoy delicious and nutritious meals without sacrificing time or flavor. With commitment, consistency, and a little creativity, you can master the art of quick cooking and maintain better control over your diabetes management.

Raw Food Diet:

Definition:

The raw food diet is based on the belief that consuming foods in their natural, uncooked state provides maximum nutritional benefits and enzymes that are destroyed during cooking. This diet typically includes raw fruits, vegetables, nuts, seeds, sprouted grains, and legumes, as well as some raw or minimally processed dairy products, eggs, fish, and meat. The raw food diet is high in vitamins, minerals, fiber, and antioxidants, and proponents believe it can lead to improved digestion, increased energy, weight loss, and reduced risk of chronic diseases.

Ingredients:

- Raw Fruits: Berries, apples, oranges, bananas, mangoes, etc.

- Raw Vegetables: Leafy greens, carrots, cucumbers, bell peppers, tomatoes, etc.

- Nuts and Seeds: Almonds, walnuts, cashews, sunflower seeds, chia seeds, flaxseeds, etc.

- Sprouted Grains and Legumes: Sprouted quinoa, lentils, chickpeas, mung beans, etc.

- Raw Dairy and Eggs (if consumed): Raw milk, cheese, yogurt, eggs (in moderation).

- Raw or Minimally Processed Meat and Fish (if consumed): Sashimi, ceviche, carpaccio, etc.

- Cold-Pressed Oils: Olive oil, coconut oil, flaxseed oil, etc.

Instructions/How to Prepare:

1. Base meals around raw fruits, vegetables, nuts, seeds, sprouted grains, and legumes.

2. Incorporate a variety of colorful fruits and vegetables into meals and snacks for their vitamins, minerals, and antioxidants.

3. Include nuts and seeds for healthy fats, protein, and fiber, using them in salads, smoothies, or raw energy bars.

4. Experiment with sprouted grains and legumes, which are easier to digest and may have increased nutrient bioavailability.

5. Be cautious with raw dairy and eggs, choosing high-quality, pasteurized options to reduce the risk of foodborne illness.

6. If consuming raw meat or fish, ensure it is fresh, high-quality, and properly handled to minimize the risk of foodborne pathogens.

7. Use cold-pressed oils like olive oil, coconut oil, and flaxseed oil for dressing salads or adding flavor to dishes.

8. Be creative with food preparation techniques such as blending, juicing, dehydrating, and marinating to enhance flavor and texture.

9. Be mindful of food safety practices when handling raw foods, including washing produce thoroughly and storing perishable items properly.

10. Listen to your body and adjust the raw food diet to meet your individual nutritional needs, and consider consulting with a healthcare professional or registered dietitian for personalized guidance and support.

Zone Diet:

Definition:

The Zone Diet is a low-glycemic, moderate-protein, and moderate-fat eating plan designed to optimize hormone levels, promote weight loss, and improve overall health and performance. It aims to balance macronutrients in a specific ratio to control inflammation, stabilize blood sugar levels, and enhance metabolic function. The diet emphasizes portion control and consuming meals that are rich in protein, low in carbohydrates, and include healthy fats to maintain a state of "the zone," where the body efficiently burns fat for fuel.

Ingredients:

- Lean Proteins: Skinless poultry, fish, seafood, tofu, tempeh, lean cuts of beef or pork.

- Non-Starchy Vegetables: Leafy greens, broccoli, cauliflower, bell peppers, zucchini, spinach, etc.

- Healthy Fats: Olive oil, avocado, nuts, seeds, fatty fish (salmon, mackerel, sardines).

- Low-Glycemic Carbohydrates (in moderation): Berries, apples, oranges, quinoa, brown rice, sweet potatoes.

- Some Dairy Products (in moderation): Greek yogurt, cottage cheese, low-fat cheese.

Instructions/How to Prepare:

1. Divide meals into specific portions of protein, carbohydrates, and fats to achieve the desired macronutrient ratio (40% carbohydrates, 30% protein, 30% fat).

2. Base meals around lean proteins such as poultry, fish, seafood, tofu, and tempeh, aiming for a portion size that fits in the palm of your hand.

3. Include plenty of non-starchy vegetables like leafy greens, broccoli, cauliflower, and bell peppers to bulk up meals and add fiber and nutrients.

4. Incorporate healthy fats like olive oil, avocado, nuts, and seeds into meals for satiety and to help balance blood sugar levels.

5. Choose low-glycemic carbohydrates such as berries, apples, oranges, quinoa, brown rice, and sweet potatoes to minimize spikes in blood sugar.

6. Be mindful of portion sizes and avoid overeating, focusing on balanced meals that include a variety of food groups.

7. Include some dairy products like Greek yogurt, cottage cheese, and low-fat cheese in moderation for additional protein and calcium.

8. Plan meals and snacks ahead of time to ensure they fit within the macronutrient ratio and support your nutritional goals.

9. Stay hydrated by drinking plenty of water throughout the day to support metabolic function and overall health.

10. Monitor progress and adjust portion sizes and food choices as needed to achieve and maintain the desired balance of macronutrients, and consider consulting with a healthcare professional or registered dietitian for personalized guidance and support.

Engine 2 Diet:

Definition:

The Engine 2 Diet, developed by firefighter Rip Esselstyn, is a plant-based eating plan designed to promote heart health, weight loss, and overall well-being. It emphasizes whole, nutrient-dense, plant-based foods while minimizing or eliminating animal products, oils, processed foods, and added sugars. The diet is inspired by the idea that eating "like a firefighter" – with a focus on whole plant foods – can prevent and even reverse chronic diseases such as heart disease, diabetes, and obesity.

Ingredients:

- Whole Grains: Brown rice, quinoa, oats, barley, whole wheat pasta, whole grain bread.

- Beans and Legumes: Black beans, lentils, chickpeas, kidney beans, edamame, tofu.

- Fruits: Berries, apples, oranges, bananas, mangoes, melons, etc.

- Vegetables: Leafy greens, broccoli, cauliflower, bell peppers, carrots, onions, etc.

- Nuts and Seeds (in moderation): Almonds, walnuts, chia seeds, flaxseeds, hemp seeds, etc.

- Herbs and Spices: Basil, oregano, garlic, ginger, turmeric, cumin, etc.

Instructions/How to Prepare:

1. Base meals around whole, plant-based foods such as whole grains, beans, legumes, fruits, and vegetables.

2. Include a variety of colorful fruits and vegetables in meals and snacks for their vitamins, minerals, and antioxidants.

3. Choose whole grains like brown rice, quinoa, oats, and barley for fiber and nutrients.

4. Incorporate beans and legumes into meals for plant-based protein, fiber, and essential nutrients.

5. Limit or eliminate processed foods, oils, added sugars, and animal products from the diet.

6. Use nuts and seeds sparingly for added texture and flavor, as they are high in calories.

7. Flavor dishes with herbs and spices instead of salt or added fats to enhance taste without extra calories.

8. Experiment with plant-based cooking techniques such as steaming, sautéing, roasting, and grilling to bring out natural flavors.

9. Be mindful of portion sizes and avoid overeating, focusing on balanced meals that include a variety of food groups.

10. Stay hydrated by drinking plenty of water throughout the day, and consider incorporating regular physical activity to complement dietary changes.

CHAPTER 11

DIETS FOR DIABETES

Dr. Bernstein's Diabetes Diet:

Definition:

Dr. Richard K. Bernstein's Diabetes Diet is a low-carbohydrate eating plan specifically designed to manage blood sugar levels and improve health outcomes for individuals with diabetes, particularly type 1 diabetes. It emphasizes controlling carbohydrate intake to prevent spikes in blood sugar, achieve stable glucose levels, and reduce the need for insulin medication. The diet consists of whole, nutrient-dense foods that are low in carbohydrates but rich in protein, healthy fats, fiber, vitamins, and minerals.

Ingredients:

- Non-Starchy Vegetables: Leafy greens, broccoli, cauliflower, bell peppers, zucchini, spinach, etc.

- Lean Proteins: Chicken, turkey, fish, seafood, eggs, tofu, tempeh, lean cuts of beef or pork.

- Healthy Fats: Olive oil, avocado, nuts, seeds, fatty fish (salmon, mackerel, sardines).

- Low-Glycemic Carbohydrates (in moderation): Berries, apples, oranges, quinoa, brown rice, sweet potatoes.

- Some Dairy Products (in moderation): Greek yogurt, cottage cheese, low-fat cheese.

Instructions/How to Prepare:

1. Limit carbohydrate intake to a specific amount per meal, typically 15 grams or less for breakfast and 30 grams or less for lunch and dinner.

2. Base meals around non-starchy vegetables, which are low in carbohydrates and high in fiber, vitamins, and minerals.

3. Include lean proteins such as poultry, fish, seafood, eggs, tofu, and tempeh in each meal to help stabilize blood sugar levels and promote satiety.

4. Incorporate healthy fats like olive oil, avocado, nuts, and seeds into meals for sustained energy and to slow the absorption of carbohydrates.

5. Choose low-glycemic carbohydrates like berries, apples, oranges, quinoa, brown rice, and sweet potatoes in moderation to minimize spikes in blood sugar.

6. Be cautious with portion sizes and avoid overeating, especially with carbohydrate-rich foods.

7. Monitor blood sugar levels regularly and adjust carbohydrate intake, insulin medication, and dietary choices as needed to maintain stable glucose levels.

8. Plan meals and snacks ahead of time to ensure they fit within the carbohydrate limits and support blood sugar control.

9. Stay hydrated by drinking plenty of water throughout the day, and consider incorporating regular physical activity to improve insulin sensitivity and overall health.

10. Work closely with a healthcare professional or registered dietitian experienced in diabetes management to develop a personalized meal plan and monitor progress over time.

Carbohydrate Counting Diet:

Definition:

The Carbohydrate Counting Diet is a method used by individuals with diabetes to manage blood sugar levels by closely monitoring carbohydrate intake. It involves counting the grams of carbohydrates in foods and balancing them with insulin doses or other blood sugar-lowering medications. The diet aims to provide flexibility in food choices while maintaining stable blood sugar levels throughout the day. It's commonly used by individuals with type 1 diabetes, type 2 diabetes, or gestational diabetes.

Ingredients:

- Carbohydrate-Containing Foods: Bread, rice, pasta, cereals, fruits, starchy vegetables, dairy products, legumes, sweets, and desserts.

- Non-Starchy Vegetables: Leafy greens, broccoli, cauliflower, bell peppers, zucchini, spinach, cucumber, etc.

- Lean Proteins: Chicken, turkey, fish, seafood, eggs, tofu, tempeh, lean cuts of beef or pork.

- Healthy Fats: Olive oil, avocado, nuts, seeds, fatty fish (salmon, mackerel, sardines).

- Low-Glycemic Carbohydrates (in moderation): Berries, apples, oranges, quinoa, brown rice, sweet potatoes.

- Some Dairy Products (in moderation): Greek yogurt, cottage cheese, low-fat cheese.

Instructions/How to Prepare:

1. Determine individual carbohydrate goals based on factors such as age, weight, activity level, blood sugar targets, and insulin sensitivity.

2. Learn to identify carbohydrate-containing foods and understand portion sizes to accurately count grams of carbohydrates.

3. Monitor carbohydrate intake throughout the day by reading food labels, using carbohydrate counting apps, or referring to carbohydrate counting resources.

4. Distribute carbohydrate intake evenly across meals and snacks to help stabilize blood sugar levels throughout the day.

5. Pair carbohydrates with lean proteins, healthy fats, and fiber-rich foods to slow the absorption of glucose and minimize blood sugar spikes.

6. Be mindful of high-glycemic carbohydrates and limit their intake to prevent rapid increases in blood sugar levels.

7. Consider timing carbohydrate intake around physical activity to optimize energy levels and blood sugar management.

8. Adjust insulin doses or other blood sugar-lowering medications based on carbohydrate intake and blood sugar levels, under the guidance of a healthcare professional.

9. Monitor blood sugar levels regularly and make adjustments to carbohydrate intake, insulin doses, or medication regimens as needed to maintain stable glucose levels.

10. Work closely with a healthcare professional or registered dietitian experienced in diabetes management to develop a personalized carbohydrate counting plan and receive ongoing support and education.

Intermittent Fasting:

Definition:

Intermittent Fasting (IF) is an eating pattern that cycles between periods of fasting and eating. It doesn't prescribe specific foods to eat but rather focuses on when to eat them. There are several variations of intermittent fasting, including the 16/8 method, the 5:2 diet, alternate-day fasting, and spontaneous meal skipping. Intermittent fasting has gained popularity for its potential benefits for weight loss, improved metabolic health, and simplified eating patterns.

Instructions/How to Prepare:

1. Choose an intermittent fasting protocol that aligns with your lifestyle, preferences, and health goals.

2. In the 16/8 method, for example, you fast for 16 hours and restrict eating to an 8-hour window each day.

3. During the fasting period, consume only non-caloric beverages such as water, black coffee, or herbal tea to help control hunger and maintain hydration.

4. Plan meals and snacks to fit within the designated eating window, focusing on nutrient-dense foods to support overall health.

5. Include a variety of whole foods such as fruits, vegetables, lean proteins, healthy fats, and whole grains in meals to promote satiety and provide essential nutrients.

6. Be mindful of portion sizes and avoid overeating during the eating window to prevent excessive calorie intake.

7. Stay hydrated by drinking plenty of water throughout the fasting and eating periods to support hydration and overall well-being.

8. Listen to your body and adjust the fasting schedule as needed to accommodate changes in hunger, energy levels, and lifestyle demands.

9. Monitor progress and pay attention to how you feel physically, mentally, and emotionally while practicing intermittent fasting.

10. Consult with a healthcare professional or registered dietitian before starting intermittent fasting, especially if you have underlying health conditions or concerns about its suitability for you.

The Biggest Loser Diet:

Definition:

The Biggest Loser Diet is a weight loss program inspired by the reality TV show "The Biggest Loser," which features contestants competing to lose the most weight through diet and exercise. The diet emphasizes portion control, calorie restriction, and regular physical activity to achieve weight loss goals. It focuses on consuming lean proteins, whole grains, fruits, vegetables, and limited amounts of healthy fats while minimizing processed foods, refined sugars, and unhealthy fats.

Ingredients:

- Lean Proteins: Chicken, turkey, fish, seafood, tofu, tempeh, lean cuts of beef or pork.

- Whole Grains: Brown rice, quinoa, oats, barley, whole wheat bread, whole grain pasta.

- Fruits: Berries, apples, oranges, bananas, mangoes, melons, etc.

- Vegetables: Leafy greens, broccoli, cauliflower, bell peppers, carrots, onions, etc.

- Healthy Fats (in moderation): Avocado, nuts, seeds, olive oil.

- Low-Fat Dairy Products (in moderation): Greek yogurt, cottage cheese, skim milk.

Instructions/How to Prepare:

1. Calculate daily calorie needs based on weight loss goals, activity level, and metabolic rate.

2. Plan meals and snacks that incorporate lean proteins, whole grains, fruits, vegetables, and healthy fats within calorie limits.

3. Use portion control techniques such as measuring food portions, using smaller plates, and being mindful of serving sizes.

4. Focus on consuming nutrient-dense foods that provide essential vitamins, minerals, and antioxidants.

5. Include regular physical activity as part of the weight loss plan, incorporating a combination of cardiovascular exercise, strength training, and flexibility exercises.

6. Be mindful of fluid intake and stay hydrated by drinking plenty of water throughout the day.

7. Monitor progress by tracking food intake, exercise, and weight loss using a journal or app.

8. Practice mindful eating by paying attention to hunger and fullness cues, eating slowly, and savoring each bite.

9. Be consistent with meal planning, grocery shopping, and food preparation to support healthy eating habits.

10. Seek support from friends, family, or a weight loss group for accountability, motivation, and encouragement throughout the journey.

Weight Watchers (WW):

Definition:

Weight Watchers (WW) is a popular weight loss program that focuses on a balanced approach to eating and lifestyle changes. It assigns point values to foods based on their nutritional content, with the goal of promoting portion control, balanced nutrition, and sustainable weight loss. Participants are assigned a daily and weekly points allowance based on their age, weight, height, gender, and weight loss goals. They can choose from a wide variety of foods and are encouraged to make healthier choices, increase physical activity, and develop lifelong habits for success.

Ingredients:

- Lean Proteins: Chicken, turkey, fish, seafood, tofu, tempeh, lean cuts of beef or pork.

- Whole Grains: Brown rice, quinoa, oats, barley, whole wheat bread, whole grain pasta.

- Fruits: Berries, apples, oranges, bananas, mangoes, melons, etc.

- Vegetables: Leafy greens, broccoli, cauliflower, bell peppers, carrots, onions, etc.

- Healthy Fats: Avocado, nuts, seeds, olive oil.

- Low-Fat Dairy Products: Greek yogurt, cottage cheese, skim milk.

- Zero-Point Foods: Certain fruits, vegetables, lean proteins, and other foods with low calorie density.

Instructions/How to Prepare:

1. Join the Weight Watchers program to access personalized support, resources, and tools for weight loss success.

2. Attend group meetings, workshops, or virtual sessions for guidance, accountability, and motivation.

3. Calculate daily and weekly SmartPoints allowance based on individual factors and weight loss goals.

4. Track food intake and activity using the WW app or website, assigning point values to foods and staying within the allotted points allowance.

5. Make healthier food choices by selecting foods that are lower in points and higher in nutritional value, such as lean proteins, whole grains, fruits, and vegetables.

6. Incorporate zero-point foods into meals and snacks to increase satiety and reduce overall calorie intake.

7. Practice portion control and mindful eating by paying attention to serving sizes and eating slowly.

8. Increase physical activity by setting activity goals, incorporating regular exercise into daily routines, and finding activities that are enjoyable and sustainable.

9. Seek support from the WW community, including coaches, members, and online forums, for encouragement, advice, and inspiration.

10. Celebrate successes, track progress, and stay committed to making healthy lifestyle changes for long-term weight management and overall well-being.

The Mayo Clinic Diet:

Definition:

The Mayo Clinic Diet is a weight loss and lifestyle program developed by the renowned Mayo Clinic. It focuses on making long-term, sustainable changes to promote healthy weight loss and improve overall health and well-being. Unlike fad diets, The Mayo Clinic Diet emphasizes practical, realistic strategies for incorporating healthy eating habits, physical activity, and positive behavior changes into daily life. The diet is divided into two phases: "Lose It!" and "Live It!" The first phase focuses on jump-starting weight loss by adopting healthy habits, while the second phase is designed to help maintain weight loss and continue making progress toward health goals.

Ingredients:

- Fruits: Berries, apples, oranges, bananas, mangoes, melons, etc.

- Vegetables: Leafy greens, broccoli, cauliflower, bell peppers, carrots, onions, etc.

- Whole Grains: Brown rice, quinoa, oats, barley, whole wheat bread, whole grain pasta.

- Lean Proteins: Chicken, turkey, fish, seafood, tofu, tempeh, lean cuts of beef or pork.

- Healthy Fats: Avocado, nuts, seeds, olive oil.

- Low-Fat Dairy Products: Greek yogurt, cottage cheese, skim milk.

Instructions/How to Prepare:

1. Set realistic weight loss and health goals based on individual preferences, needs, and medical history.

2. Adopt healthy eating habits by incorporating a variety of nutrient-rich foods such as fruits, vegetables, whole grains, lean proteins, and healthy fats into meals and snacks.

3. Focus on portion control and mindful eating by paying attention to hunger and fullness cues, eating slowly, and savoring each bite.

4. Limit or avoid processed foods, refined sugars, unhealthy fats, and excess sodium, opting for whole, minimally processed foods whenever possible.

5. Increase physical activity by setting achievable goals, incorporating regular exercise into daily routines, and finding activities that are enjoyable and sustainable.

6. Practice self-monitoring by tracking food intake, physical activity, and progress toward health goals using a journal or app.

7. Seek support from friends, family, or a weight loss group for accountability, motivation, and encouragement throughout the journey.

8. Be patient and flexible, recognizing that weight loss and lifestyle changes take time and effort, and embracing setbacks as opportunities for learning and growth.

9. Gradually transition to the "Live It!" phase of The Mayo Clinic Diet, focusing on maintaining weight loss, continuing healthy habits, and making sustainable lifestyle changes for long-term success.

10. Celebrate successes, track progress, and stay committed to making healthy choices for lifelong health and well-being.

Jenny Craig:

Definition:

Jenny Craig is a commercial weight loss program that combines pre-packaged meals and personalized coaching to help individuals achieve their weight loss goals. The program offers a variety of meal plans tailored to different dietary preferences, including standard, vegetarian, and gluten-free options. Participants receive pre-portioned meals and snacks delivered to their homes or can pick them up at Jenny Craig centers. In addition to meal delivery, Jenny Craig provides one-on-one coaching, support tools, and online resources to help clients develop healthy habits, overcome obstacles, and achieve long-term success.

Ingredients:

- Pre-Packaged Meals: Breakfasts, lunches, dinners, and snacks formulated to meet specific calorie and nutritional targets.

- Variety of Foods: Jenny Craig meals include a range of options such as pasta dishes, pizzas, burgers, soups, salads, and desserts.

- Fresh Additions: Participants are encouraged to supplement Jenny Craig meals with fresh fruits, vegetables, and dairy for added nutrition and variety.

- Snacks: Jenny Craig provides snacks such as bars, shakes, and cookies to help curb hunger between meals.

- Flexibility: Jenny Craig offers flexibility with "Your List," allowing participants to incorporate their favorite foods into their meal plans in moderation.

Instructions/How to Prepare:

1. Enroll in the Jenny Craig program and choose a meal plan based on individual weight loss goals, dietary preferences, and lifestyle.

2. Receive pre-packaged meals and snacks delivered to your home or pick them up at a Jenny Craig center, following the meal plan and eating schedule provided.

3. Enjoy Jenny Craig meals and snacks as directed, incorporating fresh fruits, vegetables, and dairy as recommended for added nutrition and variety.

4. Supplement Jenny Craig meals with water or other non-caloric beverages to stay hydrated throughout the day.

5. Schedule one-on-one coaching sessions with a Jenny Craig consultant to receive personalized support, guidance, and encouragement throughout the weight loss journey.

6. Utilize support tools such as online resources, meal planners, and the Jenny Craig app to track progress, access meal plans, and stay motivated.

7. Incorporate physical activity into daily routines to complement Jenny Craig's weight loss program and promote overall health and well-being.

8. Practice portion control and mindful eating by savoring each bite and paying attention to hunger and fullness cues.

9. Monitor weight loss progress and adjust meal plans as needed to achieve and maintain desired results.

10.   Continue following Jenny Craig's maintenance plan and lifestyle recommendations to sustain weight loss and promote long-term success.

SlimFast Diet:

Definition:

The SlimFast Diet is a popular commercial weight loss program that revolves around meal replacement shakes, bars, and snacks. It offers a structured plan designed to help individuals lose weight by replacing two meals a day with SlimFast products and enjoying one sensible meal and three low-calorie snacks. The program provides portion-controlled, calorie-controlled meals and encourages participants to follow a balanced diet, incorporating fruits, vegetables, lean proteins, and whole grains alongside SlimFast products. Additionally, SlimFast offers support tools, online resources, and a community for motivation and accountability.

Ingredients:

- SlimFast Shakes: Meal replacement shakes available in various flavors, formulated to provide essential nutrients and promote satiety.

- SlimFast Bars: Meal replacement bars available in different flavors, offering a convenient and portable option for on-the-go nutrition.

- SlimFast Snacks: Low-calorie snacks such as snack bars, chips, and crisps designed to satisfy hunger between meals.

Instructions/How to Prepare:

1. Choose a SlimFast plan based on individual weight loss goals, dietary preferences, and lifestyle.

2. Replace two meals a day with SlimFast shakes or bars, enjoying one sensible meal and three low-calorie snacks.

3. Follow the SlimFast meal plan and eating schedule, incorporating fruits, vegetables, lean proteins, and whole grains into sensible meals and snacks.

4. Drink plenty of water throughout the day to stay hydrated and promote overall health and well-being.

5. Utilize support tools such as online resources, meal planners, and the SlimFast app to track progress, access meal plans, and stay motivated.

6. Incorporate physical activity into daily routines to complement the SlimFast weight loss program and promote overall fitness and well-being.

7. Practice portion control and mindful eating by paying attention to hunger and fullness cues and savoring each bite.

8. Monitor weight loss progress and adjust meal plans as needed to achieve and maintain desired results.

9. Continue following the SlimFast maintenance plan and lifestyle recommendations to sustain weight loss and promote long-term success.

10. Seek support from the SlimFast community, including counselors, fellow participants, and online forums, for motivation, encouragement, and accountability throughout the weight loss journey.

Volumetrics Diet:

Definition:

The Volumetrics Diet, developed by Barbara Rolls, PhD, emphasizes eating high-volume, low-calorie foods to promote satiety and weight loss. It focuses on consuming foods that are low in energy density (calories per gram) but high in volume, such as fruits, vegetables, whole grains, and lean proteins. By emphasizing foods with high water content, fiber, and nutrients, the Volumetrics Diet aims to help individuals feel full and satisfied while consuming fewer calories. The diet offers flexibility and variety, allowing participants to enjoy a wide range of foods while still achieving weight loss goals.

Ingredients:

- Fruits: Berries, apples, oranges, bananas, mangoes, melons, etc.

- Vegetables: Leafy greens, broccoli, cauliflower, bell peppers, carrots, onions, etc.

- Whole Grains: Brown rice, quinoa, oats, barley, whole wheat bread, whole grain pasta.

- Lean Proteins: Chicken, turkey, fish, seafood, tofu, tempeh, lean cuts of beef or pork.

- Healthy Fats: Avocado, nuts, seeds, olive oil.

- Low-Calorie Foods: Soups, salads, broth-based dishes, fruits, vegetables, and foods with high water content and low energy density.

Instructions/How to Prepare:

1. Familiarize yourself with the concept of energy density and how it influences food choices and portion sizes.

2. Focus on consuming foods that are low in energy density, such as fruits, vegetables, whole grains, and lean proteins, as the foundation of meals and snacks.

3. Prioritize water-rich foods like soups, salads, and broth-based dishes to increase meal volume without adding extra calories.

4. Incorporate fiber-rich foods such as fruits, vegetables, whole grains, and legumes to promote satiety and support digestive health.

5. Use portion control techniques such as measuring food portions, using smaller plates, and being mindful of serving sizes to manage calorie intake.

6. Be strategic with meal planning and food choices, opting for nutrient-dense foods that provide essential vitamins, minerals, and antioxidants.

7. Include a variety of flavors, textures, and colors in meals to enhance satisfaction and enjoyment.

8. Practice mindful eating by paying attention to hunger and fullness cues, eating slowly, and savoring each bite.

9. Stay hydrated by drinking plenty of water throughout the day, as thirst can sometimes be mistaken for hunger.

10. Monitor weight loss progress and adjust meal plans as needed to achieve and maintain desired results while incorporating lifelong habits for long-term health and well-being.

SparkPeople Diet:

Definition:

The SparkPeople Diet is an online weight loss and wellness program that offers tools, resources, and support for individuals looking to achieve their health and fitness goals. The program provides personalized meal plans, workout routines, tracking tools, and a supportive community to help participants make sustainable lifestyle changes. The SparkPeople Diet focuses on a balanced approach to nutrition, exercise, and behavior change, emphasizing portion control, mindful eating, and regular physical activity. It encourages participants to set realistic goals, track progress, and celebrate successes along the way.

Ingredients:

- Balanced Meals: SparkPeople provides personalized meal plans tailored to individual dietary preferences, calorie needs, and weight loss goals.

- Nutrient-Dense Foods: Participants are encouraged to incorporate a variety of fruits, vegetables, whole grains, lean proteins, and healthy fats into their meals and snacks.

- Portion Control: SparkPeople emphasizes portion control techniques such as measuring food portions, using smaller plates, and being mindful of serving sizes to manage calorie intake.

- Exercise Routines: SparkPeople offers workout routines and fitness videos for participants to incorporate regular physical activity into their daily routines.

- Tracking Tools: SparkPeople provides tracking tools for food intake, exercise, weight loss progress, and other health metrics to help participants stay accountable and monitor their success.

- Supportive Community: SparkPeople offers a supportive online community where participants can connect with others, share experiences, and receive encouragement and motivation.

Instructions/How to Prepare:

1. Sign up for the SparkPeople program and create a personalized profile, including information about dietary preferences, weight loss goals, and activity level.

2. Receive personalized meal plans, workout routines, and tracking tools based on individual needs and goals.

3. Follow the SparkPeople meal plan, incorporating a variety of nutrient-dense foods such as fruits, vegetables, whole grains, lean proteins, and healthy fats into meals and snacks.

4. Practice portion control by measuring food portions, using smaller plates, and being mindful of serving sizes to manage calorie intake.

5. Incorporate regular physical activity into daily routines, following SparkPeople workout routines and fitness videos or engaging in other forms of exercise that are enjoyable and sustainable.

6. Use SparkPeople tracking tools to monitor food intake, exercise, weight loss progress, and other health metrics, staying accountable and motivated along the way.

7. Engage with the SparkPeople community, connecting with others, sharing experiences, and receiving encouragement and support throughout the weight loss journey.

8. Be patient and consistent, recognizing that weight loss and lifestyle changes take time and effort, and celebrating successes along the way.

9. Adjust meal plans, workout routines, and goals as needed based on progress and feedback, staying flexible and adaptable to individual needs and preferences.

10. Embrace a lifelong commitment to health and wellness, incorporating healthy habits into daily life and continuing to strive for improvement and success.

Glycemic Load Diet:

Definition:

The Glycemic Load Diet focuses on managing blood sugar levels by selecting foods based on their glycemic load, which takes into account both the quality and quantity of carbohydrates in a serving of food. The diet aims to minimize blood sugar spikes and promote stable energy levels by emphasizing foods with a low glycemic load, such as fruits, vegetables, whole grains, lean proteins, and healthy fats. It encourages portion control, balanced meals, and mindful eating to support overall health and well-being.

Ingredients:

- Low-Glycemic Foods: Fruits, vegetables, whole grains, legumes, nuts, seeds, lean proteins, and healthy fats.

- High-Fiber Foods: Foods high in fiber such as fruits, vegetables, whole grains, legumes, nuts, and seeds can help slow the absorption of carbohydrates and promote satiety.

- Healthy Fats: Avocado, nuts, seeds, olive oil, fatty fish (salmon, mackerel, sardines) provide essential nutrients and help balance blood sugar levels.

- Lean Proteins: Chicken, turkey, fish, seafood, tofu, tempeh, lean cuts of beef or pork provide satiety and support muscle health.

- Portion-Controlled Carbohydrates: Portion control is emphasized to manage carbohydrate intake and prevent blood sugar spikes.

Instructions/How to Prepare:

1. Understand the concept of glycemic load and how it influences blood sugar levels and overall health.

2. Choose foods with a low glycemic load, such as fruits, vegetables, whole grains, legumes, nuts, seeds, lean proteins, and healthy fats, as the foundation of meals and snacks.

3. Emphasize high-fiber foods to promote satiety, stabilize blood sugar levels, and support digestive health.

4. Incorporate healthy fats into meals and snacks to balance blood sugar levels and promote feelings of fullness and satisfaction.

5. Include lean proteins in meals to provide essential nutrients, promote muscle health, and support satiety.

6. Practice portion control by measuring food portions, using smaller plates, and being mindful of serving sizes to manage carbohydrate intake.

7. Be mindful of meal timing and spacing to prevent blood sugar spikes and maintain stable energy levels throughout the day.

8. Monitor blood sugar levels regularly, especially for individuals with diabetes or insulin resistance, and adjust dietary choices as needed to achieve and maintain optimal blood sugar control.

9. Stay hydrated by drinking plenty of water throughout the day to support overall health and well-being.

10.   Seek guidance from a healthcare professional or registered dietitian experienced in glycemic load and blood sugar management for personalized recommendations and support.

Low-Protein Diet:

Definition:

A low-protein diet is a dietary approach that restricts the intake of protein-rich foods, often for medical reasons. It may be prescribed for individuals with certain kidney conditions, liver disease, or metabolic disorders that impair protein metabolism. The diet typically limits high-protein foods such as meat, poultry, fish, eggs, dairy products, and legumes while allowing moderate consumption of low-protein foods such as fruits, vegetables, grains, and fats. The goal of a low-protein diet is to reduce the workload on the kidneys and liver, manage symptoms, and slow the progression of underlying medical conditions.

Ingredients:

- Low-Protein Foods: Fruits, vegetables, grains, fats, and oils are typically allowed in moderate amounts on a low-protein diet.

- Limited Protein Sources: Protein-rich foods such as meat, poultry, fish, eggs, dairy products, and legumes are restricted or limited in portion size.

- Protein-Free Foods: Certain foods may be completely avoided on a low-protein diet, especially those with high protein content.

- Fluids: Adequate hydration is important on a low-protein diet, so drinking water and other low-protein beverages is encouraged.

Instructions/How to Prepare:

1. Consult with a healthcare professional or registered dietitian to determine if a low-protein diet is appropriate for your medical condition and health needs.

2. Receive personalized guidance on the recommended daily intake of protein, as well as specific dietary restrictions and allowances.

3. Identify high-protein foods to limit or avoid, including meat, poultry, fish, eggs, dairy products, and legumes.

4. Plan meals and snacks that emphasize low-protein foods such as fruits, vegetables, grains, and fats while limiting protein-rich ingredients.

5. Use portion control techniques to manage protein intake and ensure compliance with dietary recommendations.

6. Explore alternative protein sources that are lower in protein content, such as tofu, tempeh, seitan, and certain grains and vegetables.

7. Monitor symptoms and adjust dietary choices as needed based on individual tolerance and response to the low-protein diet.

8. Stay hydrated by drinking plenty of water throughout the day, as adequate fluid intake is important for kidney function and overall health.

9. Consider working with a registered dietitian experienced in medical nutrition therapy to develop a customized meal plan and receive ongoing support and guidance.

10.   Regularly follow up with healthcare providers to assess progress, monitor kidney function, and adjust dietary recommendations as needed.

The Flex Diet:

Definition:

The Flex Diet, developed by James Beckerman, MD, is a flexible and customizable approach to weight loss and healthy living. It emphasizes the importance of flexibility, balance, and individualization in dietary choices, exercise routines, and lifestyle habits. The diet encourages participants to "flex" their approach to eating and fitness based on personal preferences, goals, and lifestyle factors. It offers practical strategies for making healthier choices, incorporating physical activity, managing stress, and building sustainable habits for long-term success.

Ingredients:

- Fruits: Berries, apples, oranges, bananas, mangoes, melons, etc.

- Vegetables: Leafy greens, broccoli, cauliflower, bell peppers, carrots, onions, etc.

- Whole Grains: Brown rice, quinoa, oats, barley, whole wheat bread, whole grain pasta.

- Lean Proteins: Chicken, turkey, fish, seafood, tofu, tempeh, lean cuts of beef or pork.

- Healthy Fats: Avocado, nuts, seeds, olive oil.

- Low-Fat Dairy Products: Greek yogurt, cottage cheese, skim milk.

Instructions/How to Prepare:

1. Determine personal health and wellness goals, considering factors such as weight loss, fitness, energy levels, and overall well-being.

2. Evaluate current eating habits, exercise routines, and lifestyle behaviors to identify areas for improvement and opportunities for change.

3. Experiment with different dietary approaches, such as Mediterranean, plant-based, low-carb, or intermittent fasting, to find what works best for individual preferences and needs.

4. Focus on consuming a balanced and varied diet that includes a wide variety of nutrient-rich foods such as fruits, vegetables, whole grains, lean proteins, and healthy fats.

5. Practice portion control and mindful eating by listening to hunger and fullness cues, eating slowly, and savoring each bite.

6. Incorporate regular physical activity into daily routines, including cardiovascular exercise, strength training, flexibility exercises, and recreational activities that are enjoyable and sustainable.

7. Manage stress and prioritize self-care by practicing relaxation techniques, mindfulness, meditation, and other stress-reducing activities.

8. Be flexible and adaptable in making dietary and lifestyle changes, recognizing that progress may not always be linear and that setbacks are part of the journey.

9. Seek support from friends, family, or a health coach for accountability, encouragement, and motivation throughout the process.

10.   Embrace a lifelong commitment to health and wellness, continually reassessing goals, making adjustments as needed, and celebrating successes along the way.

Nutrisystem:

Definition:

Nutrisystem is a commercial weight loss program that offers pre-packaged meals and snacks delivered directly to customers' homes. The program aims to simplify weight loss by providing portion-controlled, calorie- and nutrient-balanced meals that require minimal preparation. Nutrisystem offers several plans tailored to different dietary preferences and weight loss goals, including basic, core, vegetarian, and diabetic-friendly options. The program also includes support tools such as counseling, online resources, and a mobile app to help participants track progress and stay motivated.

Ingredients:

- Pre-Packaged Meals: Breakfasts, lunches, dinners, and snacks formulated to meet specific calorie and nutritional targets.

- Variety of Foods: Nutrisystem meals and snacks include a range of options such as pasta dishes, pizzas, burgers, soups, salads, and desserts.

- Fruits and Vegetables: Participants are encouraged to supplement Nutrisystem meals with fresh fruits, vegetables, and salads for added fiber, vitamins, and minerals.

- Flex Meals: Nutrisystem offers flexibility with "flex meals," allowing participants to prepare their meals using guidelines provided by the program.

- Snacks: Nutrisystem provides snacks such as bars, shakes, and cookies to help curb hunger between meals.

Instructions/How to Prepare:

1. Choose a Nutrisystem plan based on individual weight loss goals, dietary preferences, and budget.

2. Receive pre-packaged meals and snacks delivered to your doorstep, following the Nutrisystem meal plan and eating schedule.

3. Enjoy Nutrisystem meals and snacks as directed, incorporating fresh fruits, vegetables, and salads as recommended for added nutrition and variety.

4. Supplement Nutrisystem meals with water or other non-caloric beverages to stay hydrated throughout the day.

5. Utilize support tools such as counseling, online resources, and the Nutrisystem app to track progress, access meal plans, and receive personalized guidance and support.

6. Incorporate physical activity into daily routines to complement Nutrisystem's weight loss program and promote overall health and well-being.

7. Practice portion control and mindful eating by savoring each bite and paying attention to hunger and fullness cues.

8. Monitor weight loss progress and adjust Nutrisystem meal plans as needed to achieve and maintain desired results.

9. Continue following Nutrisystem's maintenance plan and lifestyle recommendations to sustain weight loss and promote long-term success.

10. Seek support from the Nutrisystem community, including counselors, fellow participants, and online forums, for motivation, encouragement, and accountability throughout the weight loss journey.

Specific Carbohydrate Diet (SCD):

Definition:

The Specific Carbohydrate Diet (SCD) is a dietary regimen designed to manage certain digestive disorders, particularly inflammatory bowel diseases (IBD) such as Crohn's disease, ulcerative colitis, and celiac disease. It aims to reduce inflammation and promote healing of the gastrointestinal tract by restricting certain carbohydrates that are thought to exacerbate symptoms. The diet focuses on consuming easily digestible, nutrient-rich foods that are low in carbohydrates and free of complex sugars and starches.

Ingredients:

- Fresh Fruits: Apples, bananas, berries, melons, etc.

- Non-Starchy Vegetables: Leafy greens, carrots, cucumbers, bell peppers, squash, etc.

- Lean Proteins: Chicken, turkey, fish, eggs, tofu, tempeh, and certain cuts of beef or pork.

- Healthy Fats: Olive oil, coconut oil, avocados, nuts, seeds.

- Fermented Foods (in moderation): Yogurt, kefir, sauerkraut, kimchi.

- Certain Legumes and Beans (in limited amounts): Lentils, black beans, navy beans.

- Homemade Broths and Soups: Chicken broth, bone broth, vegetable soup.

- Natural Sweeteners (in moderation): Honey, maple syrup.

Instructions/How to Prepare:

1. Eliminate complex carbohydrates such as grains, processed foods, and sugars from the diet.

2. Base meals around fresh fruits, non-starchy vegetables, lean proteins, and healthy fats.

3. Choose easily digestible proteins such as poultry, fish, eggs, tofu, and tempeh.

4. Incorporate healthy fats like olive oil, coconut oil, avocados, nuts, and seeds into meals for satiety and energy.

5. Include fermented foods like yogurt, kefir, sauerkraut, and kimchi in moderation to support gut health and digestion.

6. Experiment with homemade broths and soups made from scratch using nutrient-rich ingredients.

7. Be cautious with certain legumes and beans, as they may cause digestive discomfort in some individuals.

8. Use natural sweeteners like honey and maple syrup sparingly, as they are allowed in moderation on the SCD.

9. Avoid processed foods, artificial additives, and preservatives, opting for whole, unprocessed foods whenever possible.

10.   Monitor symptoms and adjust the diet as needed to manage digestive issues and promote overall well-being, and consider consulting with a healthcare professional or registered dietitian for personalized guidance and support.

Here's a 31-day meal plan focusing on quick, simple, and diabetic-friendly recipes that can be prepared in 15 minutes or less:

CHAPTER 12
31 DAY MEAL PLAN

Week 1:

Day 1:

- Breakfast: Whole grain toast with avocado slices and a boiled egg

- Lunch: Turkey and cheese roll-ups with carrot sticks

- Dinner: Lemon herb grilled chicken with steamed broccoli

Day 2:

- Breakfast: Greek yogurt with mixed berries and a sprinkle of almonds

- Lunch: Spinach and feta stuffed chicken breast

- Dinner: Stir-fried shrimp with mixed vegetables

Day 3:

- Breakfast: Smoothie made with spinach, banana, and unsweetened almond milk

- Lunch: Tuna salad lettuce wraps with cucumber slices

- Dinner: Baked salmon with roasted asparagus

Day 4:

- Breakfast: Oatmeal topped with sliced strawberries and a drizzle of honey

- Lunch: Grilled chicken Caesar salad with a light dressing

- Dinner: Turkey chili with a side of whole grain bread

Day 5:

- Breakfast: Cottage cheese with sliced peaches and a sprinkle of cinnamon

- Lunch: Quinoa and black bean salad with diced bell peppers

- Dinner: Beef stir-fry with broccoli and brown rice

Day 6:

- Breakfast: Whole grain cereal with unsweetened almond milk

- Lunch: Caprese salad with grilled chicken

- Dinner: Baked cod with sautéed spinach

Day 7:

- Breakfast: Scrambled eggs with diced bell peppers and onions

- Lunch: Turkey lettuce wraps with sliced avocado

- Dinner: Vegetable stir-fry with tofu and quinoa

Week 2:

Day 8:

- Breakfast: Whole grain toast with almond butter and sliced banana

- Lunch: Chicken and vegetable stir-fry with brown rice

- Dinner: Grilled shrimp skewers with a side of mixed greens

Day 9:

- Breakfast: Yogurt parfait with granola and mixed berries

- Lunch: Turkey and cheese wrap with lettuce and tomato

- Dinner: Lemon garlic baked chicken thighs with steamed green beans

Day 10:

- Breakfast: Smoothie bowl topped with granola, sliced apple, and cinnamon

- Lunch: Greek salad with grilled salmon

- Dinner: Stir-fried tofu with snap peas and quinoa

Day 11:

- Breakfast: Whole grain English muffin with scrambled eggs and spinach

- Lunch: Chicken Caesar salad with a light dressing

- Dinner: Turkey meatballs in marinara sauce with zucchini noodles

Day 12:

- Breakfast: Cottage cheese with pineapple chunks and a sprinkle of coconut flakes

- Lunch: Quinoa salad with chickpeas, cherry tomatoes, and feta cheese

- Dinner: Beef and broccoli stir-fry with brown rice

Day 13:

- Breakfast: Oatmeal with sliced peaches and a drizzle of maple syrup

- Lunch: Tuna salad stuffed in a whole wheat pita pocket

- Dinner: Grilled lemon herb tilapia with roasted Brussels sprouts

Day 14:

- Breakfast: Smoothie made with kale, banana, and unsweetened almond milk

- Lunch: Spinach and feta stuffed chicken breast

- Dinner: Vegetable curry with tofu and cauliflower rice

Week 3:

Day 15:

- Breakfast: Whole grain toast with mashed avocado and tomato slices

- Lunch: Turkey and cheese roll-ups with cucumber slices

- Dinner: Baked salmon with steamed broccoli

Day 16:

- Breakfast: Greek yogurt with sliced strawberries and a drizzle of honey

- Lunch: Chicken and vegetable stir-fry with quinoa

- Dinner: Grilled shrimp skewers with a side of mixed greens

Day 17:

- Breakfast: Smoothie bowl topped with sliced banana, chia seeds, and almond slices

- Lunch: Turkey and avocado wrap with lettuce and tomato

- Dinner: Lemon garlic baked chicken thighs with steamed green beans

Day 18:

- Breakfast: Whole grain cereal with unsweetened almond milk

- Lunch: Greek salad with grilled chicken

- Dinner: Stir-fried tofu with mixed vegetables and brown rice

Day 19:

- Breakfast: Cottage cheese with sliced peaches and a sprinkle of cinnamon

- Lunch: Quinoa and black bean salad with diced bell peppers

- Dinner: Beef and broccoli stir-fry with quinoa

Day 20:

- Breakfast: Oatmeal with blueberries and a drizzle of maple syrup

- Lunch: Tuna salad lettuce wraps with carrot sticks

- Dinner: Grilled lemon herb tilapia with roasted asparagus

Day 21:

- Breakfast: Scrambled eggs with diced bell peppers and onions

- Lunch: Turkey lettuce wraps with sliced avocado

- Dinner: Vegetable stir-fry with tofu and cauliflower rice

Week 4:

Day 22:

- Breakfast: Whole grain toast with almond butter and sliced banana

- Lunch: Chicken Caesar salad with a light dressing

- Dinner: Turkey meatballs in marinara sauce with zucchini noodles

Day 23:

- Breakfast: Yogurt parfait with granola and mixed berries

- Lunch: Spinach and feta stuffed chicken breast

- Dinner: Beef and vegetable stir-fry with brown rice

Day 24:

- Breakfast: Smoothie made with spinach, pineapple, and unsweetened almond milk

- Lunch: Turkey and cheese wrap with lettuce and tomato

- Dinner: Baked salmon with steamed broccoli

Day 25:

- Breakfast: Whole grain English muffin with scrambled eggs and spinach

- Lunch: Chicken and vegetable stir-fry with quinoa

- Dinner: Grilled shrimp skewers with a side of mixed greens

Day 26:

- Breakfast: Cottage cheese with sliced peaches and a sprinkle of cinnamon
- Lunch: Turkey and avocado wrap with cucumber slices
- Dinner: Lemon garlic baked chicken thighs with steamed green beans

Day 27:

- Breakfast: Oatmeal with sliced strawberries and a drizzle of honey
- Lunch: Greek salad with grilled chicken
- Dinner: Stir-fried tofu with mixed vegetables and brown rice

Day 28:

- Breakfast: Smoothie bowl topped with sliced banana, chia seeds, and almond slices
- Lunch: Turkey and cheese roll-ups with carrot sticks
- Dinner: Baked salmon with roasted Brussels sprouts

Day 29:

- Breakfast: Whole grain cereal with unsweetened almond milk
- Lunch: Tuna salad lettuce wraps with sliced avocado

- Dinner: Beef and broccoli stir-fry with quinoa

Day 30:

- Breakfast: Greek yogurt with mixed berries and a sprinkle of almonds

- Lunch: Chicken Caesar salad with a light dressing

- Dinner: Grilled lemon herb tilapia with roasted asparagus

Day 31:

- Breakfast: Scrambled eggs with diced bell peppers and onions

- Lunch: Turkey lettuce wraps with sliced tomato

- Dinner: Vegetable stir-fry with tofu and cauliflower rice

THE END

www.ingramcontent.com/pod-product-compliance
Lightning Source LLC
Chambersburg PA
CBHW081548250726
48653CB00009B/3332